The Safe Exercise Handbook

Fifth Edition

Toni Tickel Branner, M.A.
Exercise Physiologist—Professional Speaker—
Wellness Consultant
www.tonibranner.com

Illustrations by George Goebel
Photographs by Debra Young

KENDALL/HUNT PUBLISHING COMPANY
4050 Westmark Drive Dubuque, Iowa 52002

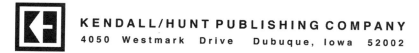

Food Article from newspaper
or
E.C. 9-22-10 :What kinds of foods contain mono-unsaturated P. 47

Contents

Preface

A healthy lifestyle is a choice. Each of us can live longer and better—if we make the decision and make a strong commitment! True wellness comes from within. We all know we should exercise and eat right but exactly how do we accomplish this? We want results in a short amount of time and we definitely do not want to become injured. *The Safe Exercise Handbook* was created to give the "how to" information in plain, basic language. Many of the fitness books on the market have good information but still include questionable stretches and calisthenics which may contribute to low back and knee problems as well as increase the risk of injury. This book promotes the importance of a regular exercise program as a means of improving your health and quality of life. A very conservative approach is utilized to assist you in designing a total workout which will accomplish your individual goals while decreasing the chance that an injury will occur.

Objectives of *The Safe Exercise Handbook*

Dispels the "no pain, no gain" and "more is better" philosophy. Exercise should not hurt!

Updates the public on current research and new concepts relating to stretching safety, proper progression, warm-up, and effective exercise methods.

Promotes total wellness. Information is provided on eating for an active lifestyle, aging with style, managing life's stressors and increasing compliance to healthy behaviors.

Provides the average person (YES! Even Couch Potatoes!) with the complete information necessary to carry out a safe, effective exercise program without burdening the reader with extraneous information. Most fitness books include very comprehensive material but the novice loses the "how to" information in the midst of scientific studies and complicated charts.

Target Audience

General Fitness Guide for Everyone: Everyone should exercise but may not be sure exactly what to do. Over 80% of Americans will eventually experience low back pain. Exercise physiologists and physical therapists now agree that all exercisers should be put on a preventive fitness program in order to avoid chronic damage to the back and other joints. Using *The Safe Exercise Handbook* as a guide, one can achieve all the benefits of regular activity while virtually eliminating the risks.

Undergraduate Fitness Classes: Used successfully for over 15 years as a text for college students enrolled in wellness-oriented activity classes (aerobic dance, exercise and conditioning, weight training, jogging, walking, water exercise, and others).

Worksite Fitness and Wellness Programs: Designed as follow-up for exercise testing and health risk appraisal in supervised wellness programs. Forms for recording results of health and fitness screening as well as space for individual exercise programs and daily fitness logs are included.

School Resource for Educators: Used successfully to introduce teachers and administrators to new concepts in exercise and health. Also appropriate as a text for senior high students.

Patient Education for Physicians, Physical Therapists, Registered Dieticians, Nurses, Health Educators, and Personal Trainers: Do not just tell patients to exercise. Tell them exactly what to do! Recommend exercise to your patients with very specific guidelines. *The Safe Exercise Handbook* is a complete, inexpensive guide to starting a conservative fitness program. Space is included to write individual instructions and modifications.

Acknowledgments

This book was created to fill a special need. When I was hired to implement the Employee Health and Fitness Center at the University of North Carolina, I received encouragement from faculty and staff who said they no longer hurt after exercise sessions prescribed by our staff and they were seeing results for the first time. The time demands of individual counseling prompted the creation of this manual so that each participant would have all of the information to take home with them (and pictures of the exercises!). Credit must be extended to these dedicated employees.

Thanks also to the faculty and staff at UNC-Chapel Hill, my college students who are so enthusiastic and interested in wellness and exercise, and my private clients who continue to remind me that safer is better. A special acknowledgement to the thousands of school administrators, teachers, and staff who have allowed me to disperse this information into the school system. The health of our educators and our children is the key to a future of wellness.

Each day I am inspired and energized by the participants in the MACFit program at the Mecklenburg Aquatic Club in Charlotte, North Carolina. During my years as Fitness Director I have had the opportunity to put research into practice. Our participants report disappearing back pain, successful weight control, decreased blood pressure, better control of diabetes, and more energy for the fun things in life. Observing eighty year olds lifting weights, gaining muscle mass, and looking decades younger than they are takes away my fear of aging.

A special thank you to Fitness Wholesale, the company that provides the wonderful exercise bands included with this book. They have always provided the highest quality equipment and resources for my clients and have always included *The Safe Exercise Handbook* in their catalog.

Currently, there is an overwhelming and confusing amount of fitness, nutrition, and health information available to everyone in the print world, the internet, and on TV. In light of this I decided to develop a service for my clients to help them sort and interpret the important research. After 20 years of professional speaking and wellness consulting on my own, I decided to develop a team of professionals and motivators who truly care about the health of others. Our Wellness From Within Team provides seminars on many topics and a free email newsletter to give practical up-to-date advice to our busy clients. Write me to get on our subscription list (tonibranner@aol.com). Be sure to mention any special health concerns or areas of interest. Thank you to Terry Hauser, Genia Rogers,

Terrie Reeves and the rest of our team who have worked hard to make this dream a reality.

The basic philosophy and inspiration for *The Safe Exercise Handbook* must be credited to my mother, Rebecca Henley Brown. After teaching fitness and aerobic dance classes in our basement and at a local health spa for many years, she enrolled at George Mason University to earn a B.S. in exercise science. Her business, The Exercise Studio, Inc. evolved, providing safe, effective classes which were years ahead of the rest of the fitness world. Innovations in low-impact aerobic dance, intensive instructor training, and modifying for individual differences were a part of her program long before the information appeared in exercise books. She was in the very first group to earn official certification as an exercise leader. As I entered the health field I was amazed at how many ineffective and contraindicated exercises were still a regular part of most fitness regimes. *The Safe Exercise Handbook,* in this fifth edition, strives to reeducate this population and to show newcomers the way to lifetime, injury-free fitness.

My husband Billy is my soul-mate and always supports my efforts to put my passion for helping people into practice. Thank you to my beautiful and sweet children, Jenna and Will, who inspired me to write a children's book to make this same information available to the very young. *Wilby's Fitness Book* is an innovative, rhyming, story book for children that teaches specific fitness skills, nutrition, and self-esteem. The next generation does not have to experience the difficulties that we have encountered. Exercise and eating right could and should be second nature to them!

And finally, thank you for taking time to care about your health. Enjoy!

Introduction

SEE The Way to a Healthier Lifestyle

Safety

Effectiveness

Efficiency

Safety: Most things seem to evolve or change over time, hopefully for the better. The same is true for exercise. Professionals are realizing that some of the activities, stretches, and calisthenics that we have always done may be causing chronic or acute injuries. The new philosophy in health and fitness focuses on achieving the benefits without taking on the associated risks. Although all risks cannot be eliminated, most individuals should be able to participate in a fitness routine without experiencing injury, pain or discomfort and should be able to continue this program for a lifetime. This concept is difficult for those who adhere to the "no pain, no gain" and the "more is better" philosophy.

Choosing the safest and most effective fitness program should be the primary goal for all individuals who wish to exercise. The problems arise when people choose the older and less safe methods for the sake of tradition or simply out of habit. We now know that some of our favorite stretches and exercises are not very safe and in some cases are not very effective. Some of these may not cause discomfort initially, but over time may lead to chronic, overuse injuries. The secret to exercising safely is moderation. Do enough to achieve the benefits without creating unnecessary stress or injury. Another key element is knowledge. The more you know about exercise principles and proper technique, the more effective and more rewarding your workout will be.

Also remember that exercising for health is much different than training for athletics. Often athletes risk injury for the sake of competition or recreation. Dancers and gymnasts place their bodies in extreme positions for competitive reasons and to create artistic images. If your goal is to live longer and be fit and healthy, there is no need to do anything which jeopardizes your body. Exercise does not have to be painful. If it hurts, leave it out! Seek help from a professional to find a safe alternative.

Effectiveness: Every exercise should have a purpose with a specific outcome in mind and the benefit should always outweigh the risk. Using the proper frequency, intensity, and duration is the key to making sure you accomplish your goals.

Efficiency: In these busy times it is important that we not waste minutes on movement that does not help us accomplish our goals. If you have a limited amount of time to devote to exercise you want to make the most of this time. For example, when strengthening biceps it will save you time to work two arms at once.

Medical Considerations

This book promotes the importance of a regular exercise program as a means of improving your health and quality of life. A conservative approach is utilized to assist you in designing a total workout which will accomplish your individual goals while decreasing the chance that an injury will occur. A book cannot replace personal guidance from a trained exercise professional. When you have questions seek information or classes in your community: at local YMCA's, private gyms, colleges, universities, and from certified personal trainers.

Before embarking on any fitness program you should consider a medical evaluation of your current health status. If you have been following a regular exercise routine or if you are under 35 years of age and have no significant health problems it is okay to begin a moderate exercise program and progress slowly. If, however, you have a medical problem, have never exercised, or are over 35 it is imperative that you consult with your physician concerning any special needs or contraindications.

Sticking With It! Exercise Adherence

It is relatively easy to start a program, sticking with it long enough to gain benefits and to form a habit is difficult for most people. Here are some suggestions and tips to help you adhere to your healthy lifestyle changes.

Pick activities that appeal to you. Your program should be varied enough to maintain interest and diminish boredom. Your chosen activities should reflect your objectives, time available, and personal style.

Remember that exercise is not always fun or convenient. Your workout must become a habit, just like brushing your teeth. And of course, you always feel better afterwards.

Make it as convenient as possible. If you have to drive twenty miles to exercise you are less likely to do it than if you can stop on the way home from work.

Have an alternate plan for vacations, weekends, rainy days, or very busy times.

Utilize support systems. A friend, co-worker, or spouse can cover responsibilities for you while you exercise and you can do the same for them. An exercise partner or class may hold you accountable to your commitment.

If it hurts—stop! You are unlikely to continue any activity which is painful or causes delayed muscle soreness. Seek professional advice and switch to a different activity until the injury heals.

Keep a log or journal (see appendix) of your activity or note workouts in your calendar. It is motivating to look back on our accomplishments and to see progress. A written six week contract with yourself has also been shown to be helpful.

Do not try too much too soon. It can be overwhelming to start exercising, change your diet, and quit smoking all at the same time. I recommend starting with exercise. As your energy increases and you feel better you will be motivated to begin new lifestyle changes.

Avoid boredom, vary your workout. Try different activities, locations, and exercise partners. Make exercise a family affair. Weekend hikes, cycling trips and nature walks are wonderful.

You will have bad days and bad weeks. If you miss an exercise session, eat a banana split, or smoke a cigarette, remember that it is not the end of your healthy lifestyle plan. Analyze why it happened, admit that you need to do better next week, and get back on target.

Reward your efforts. If you stick with your plan for three months reward yourself with a new outfit, tennis racquet, or weekend trip. Or you can give yourself a well deserved pat on the back!

Remember.......
If you cannot afford prevention....
(time/money/effort)
how will you afford disease?

Chapter One

THE BENEFITS OF EXERCISE

Hundreds of scientific and practical experiments have been carried out in an attempt to pinpoint the benefits of regular exercise. Some of the information is conflicting but overall the data suggests that being fit can have a positive impact on many aspects of your life. Most important is to act now. Just because you were active earlier in your life does not mean you are immune from the effects of a sedentary lifestyle. The evidence is too great. You can put off cleaning out your closet or weeding the flowers but you cannot afford to procrastinate with regard to fitness any longer. It is never too late to start.

The list below highlights some of the well researched benefits of exercise. Most of the benefits are related to aerobic exercise, strength training, and stretching, however, people who are generally active in daily living will experience some of the same results. Recent studies have demonstrated that moderate activity is almost as beneficial as strenuous, high-intensity exercise in preventing heart disease and increasing longevity. You don't have to run marathons to receive the benefits.

It is important to engage in activities which are fun and enjoyable. Modest amounts of physical activity, such as climbing stairs, mowing the grass, and walking the golf course (or your dog) will have a positive impact on health.

Physiological Benefits of Regular Aerobic Exercise

1. **Decreased Risk of Coronary Heart Disease(CHD)** - CHD is caused by a lack of blood supply to the heart muscle, resulting from a degenerative disorder called atherosclerosis. Buildup of plaque and fat on the lining of arteries begins in early childhood. Active kids become active adults and physical activity reduces the risk of blockage. Regular exercisers add quality and years to their life. If a heart attack does occur, regular exercisers have less chance of a fatal or recurring event.

2. **Reduced Hypertension** - Hypertension is abnormally high blood pressure. It is especially prevalent among African-Americans. Aerobic and muscular exercise has been found to decrease elevated systolic and diastolic blood pressure.

3. **Improved Blood Lipids and Lipoproteins** - Exercise has been shown to effectively reduce triglycerides, total cholesterol and LDL cholesterol all of which are related to a higher incidence of coronary artery disease (blockage of arteries which can lead to chest pain and/or heart attack). HDL cholesterol, a beneficial type of cholesterol which helps clear the arteries, is usually increased. Therefore, regular aerobic exercise combined with a low-fat/high-fiber diet can reduce the buildup of the plaque which causes blockage in arteries.

4. **Enhanced Cardiac Function** - Exercise makes the cardiorespiratory system stronger and more efficient. Specific changes include:

    • Lower resting heart rate (this means your heart has to beat fewer times per minute to supply your body with adequate oxygen and nutrients).

    • Increased stroke volume (the amount of blood pumped by the heart with each beat is increased)

    • Higher oxygen uptake (Since your heart can pump more blood per beat, your body's capacity to consume oxygen during exercise is enhanced. The greater volume of blood, and therefore oxygen, delivered to the muscle cells results in increased stamina)

    • Increased metabolism of fat and carbohydrate (trained muscle cells are more efficient at utilizing fat due to increased blood flow and the greater activity of fat-metabolizing enzymes. The muscle cells can also store more glycogen which makes more carbohydrate available for use).

5. **Enhanced Bone Health** - Weight-bearing exercise such as recreational jogging, aerobic dancing, brisk walking, and cycling for the lower skeleton and weight training for the upper body can increase or maintain overall bone mass. Inactivity, on the other hand, contributes to calcium loss from the bones and to osteoporosis. Regular weight-bearing activity begun at an early age combined with proper nutrition, adequate calcium, and possible estrogen replacement therapy after menopause can have a positive effect on lifelong bone health.

6. **Lower Smoking Risk** - Exercisers are less likely to smoke than sedentary people. For those who do smoke, physical activity lowers the risk of coronary artery disease.

7.   **Healthier Weight and Body Fat -** Since obesity is a major risk factor for cardiovascular disease, diabetes and other health problems, reducing your risk could save your life. Lean body mass (muscle) is more metabolically active than fat which means you will burn more calories at rest.

8.   **Better Control of Blood Glucose -** Diabetics can benefit from regular physical activity combined with a proper diet and appropriate medications.

9.   **Increased Muscular Strength and Flexibility -** As we grow older strength and flexibility become a deciding factor in our ability to function in normal and necessary activities. Exercise has been shown to delay and possibly prevent some of the degenerative problems associated with aging. Muscular balance can prevent lower back injuries, knee problems, and joint problems.

Other Possible Physical Benefits Shown Through Research

Improves the function of your immune system.
Improves posture.
Helps relieve the pain of tension headaches.
Helps you to incur fewer medical and health-care expenses.
Reduces your risk for developing colon, breast, and prostate cancer.
Improves your heat tolerance.
Helps you sleep better.
Helps to relieve or prevent constipation.
Helps you adapt to cold environments.
Reduces your risk of gastrointestinal bleeding.
Reduced risk of endometriosis.
More energy to do the things you want to do!

Psychological Benefits of Regular Exercise

1.   Reduces depression

2.   Improves confidence and self-esteem

3.   Promotes a sense of well-being and positive mood

4.   Increased alertness and clearer thinking

5.   Improves ability to handle stress

6. Decreases tension

7. Improves attitude toward work and reduces missed workdays due to illness

8. Helps you to combat substance abuse

9. Helps reduce pre-menstrual tension

10. Improves overall quality of life to allow you to maintain function and take care of yourself until the day you die (at 110 years old of course!).

Chapter Two

Achieving Optimal Fitness

Develop Cardiovascular Endurance (Aerobic Fitness)

The word *aerobic* means "with oxygen". Oxygen is necessary to burn the fuels which produce energy for prolonged activity. By exercising aerobically we initiate physiologic changes which increase the efficiency of the heart, lungs, and circulatory system. A healthy heart has the ability to supply plenty of oxygen and nutrients to the working muscles during normal activities as well as any emergency situations which might arise.

Aerobic activities are those that are rhythmical, continuous, and involve large muscle groups. Aerobic activities such as walking, running, cycling, swimming, and aerobic dance increase the heart rate to a target level and maintain it at that level for a certain length of time. Chapter Four demonstrates how to choose an activity and how to determine the appropriate frequency, duration, and intensity of your cardiovascular workout.

Develop Muscular Strength and Endurance

Muscular strength is the amount of force a muscle can exert or resist for a brief period of time. Research and practical experience tell us that if we stress a muscle or muscle group more than it is normally used to, it will eventually adapt and improve its function. Therefore, certain exercises are designed to increase strength so that we may perform our everyday activities with less exertion and less chance of injury. New research tells us that muscular strengthening exercises play a key part in preventing osteoporosis and preventing decreases in metabolism. If a muscle is stressed less than it is usually accustomed it will atrophy and lose strength. Broken limbs are good examples. The limb is immobilized for a length of time and when the cast is removed, one limb is usually smaller than the other. The same thing happens when you never perform strength movements. When your muscle mass is decreased you will experience a decreased resting metabolism.

Professionals now agree that strength training is an essential part of a complete fitness program. Exercises utilizing weight training, calisthenics, and rubber bands will help to increase muscular strength.

Muscular endurance describes the ability of muscles to sustain repeated contractions or apply sustained force against a fixed object. If having muscular strength allows you to pick up a heavy box, then having muscular endurance allows you to pick up ten boxes one after the other. Activities such as sit-ups, push-ups, raking leaves, shoveling snow, and pushing a lawn mower all require prolonged muscular exertion. Chapter Five describes muscular endurance exercises which are safe and effective.

Muscular Balance

One of the most effective things one can do to improve health is to develop adequate muscular balance. Often individuals have sufficient strength in some muscle groups but are deficient in others. For example, we use our quadriceps (thigh muscles) every time we walk, run, climb stairs, etc. Our hamstrings (back of the thigh) usually receive no significant exercise during everyday activities. The strong quadriceps pulls with more force on the skeletal system, especially the hip, back, and knee. This kind of muscular imbalance is often the source of lower back pain, hip pain, knee injuries, and various other injuries. It can also affect your posture, movement patterns, and make you more prone to injuries from other reasons. Thus, when using strength training you must concentrate on these weaker muscles to create balance.

A good rule to remember is: **STRETCH THE STRONG MUSCLES AND STRENGTHEN THE WEAK ONES! IF YOU HAVE TIME DO ALL OF THEM.**

Extra Strengthening for These Muscle Groups:

Rectus Abdominus, Transverse Abdominis, and Internal and External Obliques (Abs)

Erector Spinae (lower back)

Hamstrings (back of thigh)

Abductor (outer thigh)

Rhomboids (Upper Back)

Deltoids (top of shoulders)

Triceps (back of upper arm)

Include These Muscle Groups if You Have Time and Add Extra Stretching:

Iliopsoas (hip flexors, front of hips)

Quadriceps (front of thigh)

Adductors (inner thigh)

Gastrocnemius (calf muscles)

Biceps (upper arm)

Functional Strength and Core Stabilization?

Exercises which help prepare you for real-life activities require functional training. By recreating the movement patterns you use in your daily activities you become stronger and more prepared for work and recreation. Focusing on coordination, balance, muscular control, and the speed of movements are some ways to work on functional fitness. Mimicking the actual movement when you exercise is a simple way to accomplish this. An example would be practicing the movement of picking up a heavy baby out of a car seat or unloading boxes from the trunk of your car. It is also important to evaluate how much flexibility is necessary for your specific activities and to train with that goal in mind.

Your core muscles include your abdominal muscles, your back muscles, and smaller muscles involved in posture and support of the spine. This book includes exercises which focus on keeping the core muscles stable and strong as well as increasing strength during movement. Stability balls and standing exercises are great for improving core strength. Functional training should only be used in conjunction with traditional strength training. See Chapter Five for a plan to develop functional fitness.

Develop Flexibility

Flexibility is the range of motion possible around a joint. Stretching exercises are utilized to maintain or increase this range of movement, to help prevent muscle soreness, and to prevent long-term injuries. The goal of a stretching program should be to maintain maximal function. We do not want to lose our ability to reach, tie our shoes, or drive a car. We also want to be able to enjoy life. This means maintaining joint range of motion forever. Your stretching program only takes five or ten minutes, three or more days per week. It is best performed at the end of the aerobic or muscular workout when the muscles are warm all the way to the core. It is not always necessary to stretch at the beginning of your workout. For most activities saving it for the end is best (See Chapter Three).

Since flexibility is specific to every joint, it is incorrect to refer to flexibility in a general sense (i.e. John has good flexibility). Each joint must be evaluated separately. Another common misconception is to assume that to have good flexibility a person must have an excessive amount, such as a gymnast or a dancer. Athletes and performers often place their bodies in positions which stretch muscles and connective tissue beyond the point deemed necessary for normal function. They do this for the sake of competition or aesthetics which requires special coaching and conditioning to avoid injuries.

Many people hate to stretch because they feel uncomfortable. This is because they have been using positions and techniques designed for people with high levels of flexibility and most of us are not that flexible. Some of the stretching positions we have used traditionally are now known to be injurious (or they place your body in a vulnerable position). For example, the *Hurdler's* position puts the knee in a position of misalignment which can cause injury to tendons and ligaments. The good news is that a regular stretching program can produce results, be painless, and promote relaxation and release of muscular tension. Chapter Three details contraindicated stretches and gives alternatives for safely increasing flexibility.

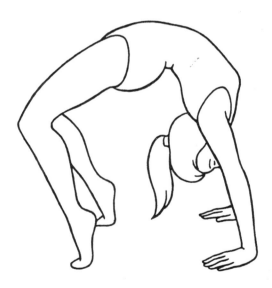

A gymnast performing a back arch. This high degree of flexibility is not necessary to function normally in every day life and may be injurious to someone who is not properly trained.

Improve or Maintain Body Composition

Your body weight includes the weight of all your muscles, bones, organs, body fluids, and body fat. If the fat is removed, all that remains is your lean body mass. Too much adipose tissue (fat) has been associated with many health risks including heart disease, diabetes, hypertension, arthritis, gall bladder disease, cirrhosis of the liver, hernia, intestinal problems, and sleep disorders. Exercise works to increase the lean body mass and decrease body fat.

Your percentage of body fat is a much better indicator of your fitness than your weight. For example, many athletes would be overweight according to typical weight charts. However, if we measured their percentage of body fat, it would probably be low or within normal ranges. There are also many thin, sedentary people who weigh very little but have a high percentage of body fat. It would be dangerous for these individuals to lose weight, they must exercise to increase their lean muscle mass. Research has demonstrated that if overweight people participate in moderate physical activity on a regular basis they will live longer than similarly overweight people who do not exercise. In plain terms this means: Even if you don't lose weight a regular exercise program will increase the quality of your life and allow you to live longer!

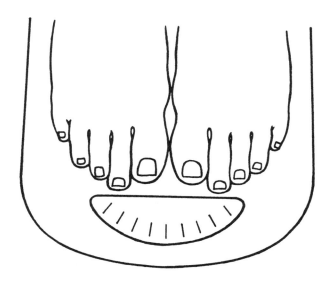

Scales may not give us all of the information needed to determine health status. The body fat percentage is often more important.

Long-term regular exercise usually decreases body fat but does not always have an immediate effect on body weight. This is because you are gaining muscle mass as you lose the fat. If you are trying to lose excess weight, do not become discouraged if your weight does not change immediately. Remember that your body composition is improving. If you can imagine the fat cells in your body just hanging our, not needing much (fuel, oxygen, etc.), not doing much—just there! Now picture your muscle cells—constantly using energy, needing huge deliveries of oxygen, and staying very busy. Because lean (muscle) tissue is more metabolically active than fat, you will burn more calories all of the time, even when you are sitting around or sleeping! Exercise also increases your ability to mobilize and oxidize fat. This enhances weight loss efforts, conserving lean body mass and preventing regain of lost body weight.

Body fat varies widely even between fit individuals. We do know that the average person in the United States tends to be over fat. Women are considered to be obese at a body fat of 32% or higher, men at 25% or higher. Women are considered to be fit at 21-24% body-fat and men at 14-17%. Females who drop below 10-13% may cease menstruating. This decreased estrogen level promotes calcium loss from the bones, increasing the risk of fractures and osteoporosis. This is a common problem for those with eating disorders, long distance runners, and other endurance athletes. Athletes also have much higher levels of oxidative stress (see Chapter 7) and therefore need even more antioxidants from fruits and vegetables than the normal population.

There are four common ways of determining body fat: Hydrostatic weighing, circumference measurements, bioelectrical impedance, and skin-fold measurements. Choose a qualified exercise physiologist to perform the test for you. A trained professional can help you keep records of your body fat over time. If you do not have access to these tests you may find that looking objectively at your physique often tells you as much as you need to know. It is important to remember that your body type and genetic background do play a part in determining your body composition. Decide what you can achieve realistically and slowly work toward your goal.

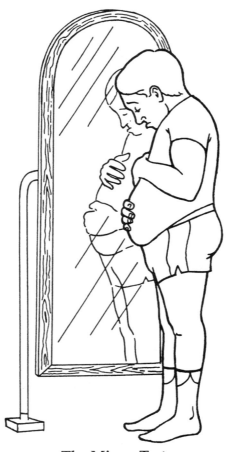

The Mirror Test

Other Required Ingredients for Optimal Fitness

- Eat Well! Make Permanent Changes

- Manage and Reduce Chronic Stress

- Stop Smoking and Protect Yourself from Secondary Smoke

- See Your Physician Regularly. Participate in All Recommended Screenings

- Get Enough Sleep and Rest

- Surround Yourself with Support: Family, Friends, and Co-Workers

- Nurture Your Spiritual Life

- Make the Most of What You Have: Focus on a Positive Self-Image

Chapter Three

WARMING-UP AND STRETCHING

Both competitive and recreational athletes often make the mistake of equating the words 'warm-up' and 'stretching.' They comprise two separate parts of your workout. Although stretching exercises can be included in the pre-workout routine, the most important goal when preparing to exercise should be to increase the body temperature and to prepare the muscles, connective tissue, and circulatory system to safely accommodate more intense exercise. **Stretching cold can be more harmful than not stretching at all.** The best time to stretch is after cardiovascular exercise or a muscular workout when the body temperature is elevated. The goal of stretching is to optimize joint range of motion but maintain stability in the joint. It is crucial to do the stretches correctly and to avoid unsafe positions.

For these reasons the warm-up phase is divided into two parts: The *circulatory (thermal) warm-up* followed by the optional *stretching warm-up.*

The Circulatory/Thermal Warm-up

The circulatory or thermal warm-up should be designed to raise local and core temperature and to increase blood flow to the working muscles. Because of this increase in temperature and blood saturation, a proper warm-up improves performance and reduces injury. Improved blood flow is necessary so that enough oxygen and nutrients are carried to the cells and so that the additional waste products produced can be adequately removed. The heart also has time to adjust to the increased demand. Studies show that beginning too quickly can cause abnormal heart rhythms. The higher body temperature allows nerve impulses to travel faster which maximizes coordination. In addition, the metabolic reactions that produce fuel for the activity occur more quickly and more efficiently. In the muscle, the mechanical efficiency of contraction is enhanced and the contraction itself is quicker and more forceful. Muscles are more elastic and the extensibility of tendons, ligaments and other connective tissue is increased.

These physiologic principles make a strong case for not omitting the thermal/circulatory warm-up. It is especially important when exercise is performed in a cool or cold environment. Extremely cold surroundings may require a ten to fifteen minute circulatory warm-up. On a summer day three minutes might be enough. If an active warm-up is not possible or convenient, a passive warm-up such as a hot shower or applied heat can also be effective.

Practically, the circulatory warm-up is simple. It is accomplished by performing rhythmical, continuous movement of medium intensity for four to six minutes. It is always a good idea to mimic some of the movements which you will be doing in your workout. Examples of proper circulatory warm-ups include:

Walking with arm movements

Slow cycling, swimming or jogging

Mild rope skipping

Low intensity, low impact aerobic dance routine

Side steps with forehand and backhand swings (without the racquet)

Remember that no stretching should be included during this segment. The circulatory warm-up should continue until a light perspiration is present. At this point you should not feel tired or out of breath. Your heart rate and respiration rate are slightly elevated, your muscles are warmer, and you are ready to proceed to the next portion of your workout.

Benefits of an Effective Warm-up

Increased body temperature

Increased heart rate, blood flow, and rate of breathing

Blood flow sent to working muscles

Increased metabolic rate (more fuel for activity)

Faster transmission of nerve impulses

Decreases chance of soreness caused by a build up of lactic acid

Increased synovial fluid in the joints

Increases speed and force of muscle contractions

Decreases risk of acute injuries to muscles and connective tissues

The Stretching Warm-up

Mild stretching exercises can follow the circulatory warm-up. The muscles are still not as warm as they should be, therefore, more intense stretching is better left for the end of the workout. Warm tissues stretch more easily, providing more permanent results and less risk of injury. There is no evidence that stretching before a workout actually prevents injuries. Research shows the best time to stretch is at the end, however, many people report that mild stretching before intense activity makes the workout more comfortable. Although athletes may require this phase, non-ballistic activities like walking, swimming and cycling may not require a stretching warm-up. Just start slowly and gradually build intensity as your body warms up. Stretching cold is worse than not stretching at all. If your time is limited, save your stretching until the end of your workout.

Final Stretch

The final stretch is the last segment of your workout and should consist of five to fifteen minutes of stretching and relaxation exercises. This will improve your flexiblity and may reduce the chance of delayed onset muscle soreness. Since your muscles and connective tissue are completely warm, it is okay to stretch using more tension than you did in the stretching warm-up. Always move slowly into the stretched position, hold at least 10 seconds and release slowly from the position. In addition to increasing or maintaining flexibility, this stretching serves as a final cool-down from the aerobic and muscular conditioning exercises. After the final stretch you should feel slightly fatigued but not exhausted. Your body temperature and heart rate should be close to your resting levels and the majority of perspiration should have evaporated.

Benefits of a Proper Stretching Program

Improved posture and body symmetry

Increased range of motion for each joint

Minimize low back pain and problems

Delay onset of muscle fatigue

Minimize soreness

Promote relaxation and reduce anxiety

Types of Stretching

Ballistic stretching consists of quick, repetitive, bouncing type movements. Although this method is somewhat effective, the increased range of motion is achieved through a series of jerks and pulls on the resistant muscle tissue. The momentum can result in damage to muscle and connective tissue and may be responsible for increased muscle soreness.

Static stretching involves gradually going into a position of stretch until tension is felt. The position is then held for ten to thirty seconds or even longer. Optimal gains have been reported with four sets of 12-18 seconds per stretch. If your time is limited, hold each stretch 10-15 seconds. Since static stretching is more controlled, there is less chance of exceeding the limits of the tissue thereby creating injury.

Dynamic stretching involves moving slowly and with control through a range of motion. You must have completed a thermal warm-up for this to be safe. For example, in a lunging calf stretch (gastrocnemius), slowly bend your back knee, lifting your heel off the floor. Now straighten the knee slowly and press the heel back into the floor. Repeat several times.

Contract and Relax methods involve contraction of muscles or muscle groups for five to ten seconds followed by relaxing and stretching. Traditionally, this procedure has been utilized by therapists for rehabilitation purposes. If carefully instructed and supervised, contract/relax methods can be effective in flexibility programs. Some of the positions require a partner, however, which increases the risk of overstretching and consequent injury.

General Rules for Stretching Safely

Avoid Extreme Hyperextension of the Spine (arching the back)-This position places the back in a vulnerable position. The disks pull away in the front and the spinal processes can grind against each other. A small amount of active and passive back extension is necessary to maintain back health. A cautious approach is necessary to avoid injury.

Avoid Locking any Joint-When stretching, performing muscular conditioning exercises, lifting weights, or any other activity it is important to keep the knees and other joints 'softened' to guard against unnecessary stretching or tearing of ligaments and connective tissue. Ligaments are not meant to be stretched (muscles and tendons can be lengthened) as this decreases stability in the joint.

Never Force a Movement-Do not place your body in unnatural positions and do not perform movements which cause discomfort. Notice signs that you may be overextending your limits. Muscles stretch best when relaxed.

Avoid Forward Flexion of the Spine-Some of the positions which result in a high injury rate involve forward flexion of the spine. Forward flexion simply means bending forward from the waist.

The spine is a flexible column formed of a series of bones called vertebrae. The vertebrae are stacked on top of each other with the spinal cord running through the middle. Between each one are intervertebral discs which are filled with a soft, pulpy, highly elastic substance. These discs act as cushions for the bony vertebrae, however, they tend to degenerate with age. Forward flexion causes the front border of the intervertebral discs to compress. Hanging forward in this position requires the disks, ligaments, and other connective tissues to bear almost all the stress. This makes the spine extremely vulnerable to injury. At 40 degrees of flexion the pressure inside the disk is doubled. This can cause pressure on the nerves which run along the spine resulting in low back aches or radiating pain. The pressure this places on the pulpy center can be so great that it eventually ruptures causing severe back pain. The problem is magnified if any twisting motion is added to the forward flexion (windmills, side bends, elbow to knee, etc.). **Over time these forward flexed positions contribute to chronic degeneration and can greatly increase the chance of low back pain or herniation of a disc. The damage occurs over many years. No symptoms of disk degeneration may appear until significant damage has already occured.**

When lifting heavy objects we are often reminded to use our legs, not our back. The justification for this is the same as for avoiding forward and side bending exercise positions. Exercise is not the only culprit. Gardening, picking up dirty socks, lifting objects incorrectly, and other forward bending movements can all contribute to wear and tear on the discs. Good News! There are many alternate stretches which will accomplish the same goal as toe touches without putting the spine in a compromised position.

Contraindicated Stretching Positions:
What To Do Instead

The positions described in this chapter are frequently used as stretching exercises. They are divided into muscle groups and are then catagorized as 'contraindicated,' 'conditional,' or 'safe.' Read this section and then use *The Five Minute Stretch* (Appendix 1) to begin your flexibility program. It is a summary of the safe positions and includes all major muscle groups.

CONTRAINDICATED

It is best to completely avoid *contraindicated* positions or stretches. Although it is not guaranteed that an injury will result, the chances are much increased and there are always safe and effective alternatives. Even if you do not feel pain while performing a contraindicated stretch, damage may be occurring which will show up later. Why take a chance if there is a safer way to accomplish the same goal?

CONDITIONAL

Some positions are not really dangerous, they are just uncomfortable and ineffective for individuals who have poor flexibility in a specific joint. These are called *conditional* exercises and should only be used if they feel comfortable and if they accomplish the desired goal for each individual.

SAFE

Safe positions can be used by almost everyone but precautions still need to be taken to insure correct form and technique.

Stretching the Neck and Shoulders

Never Hyperextend the neck -
This means you should not bend your neck to the back or do full head circles. This compresses the cervical discs and can result in acute or chronic injury.

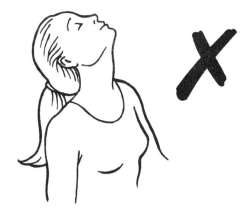

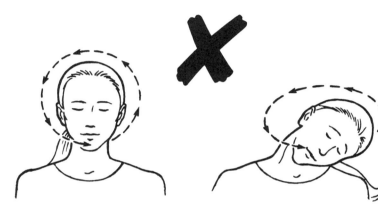

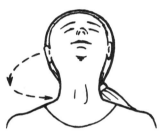

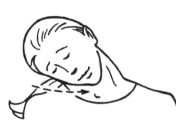

Slow, static stretches which include dropping the head to the center, turning to each side, and placing the ear to the shoulder will safely relieve tension and tightness in the neck and shoulders. Controlled half circles also help to relieve tension.

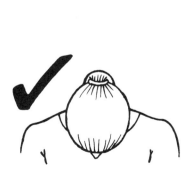

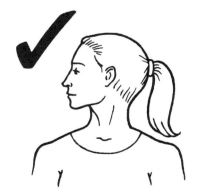

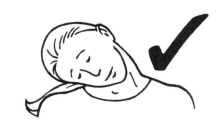

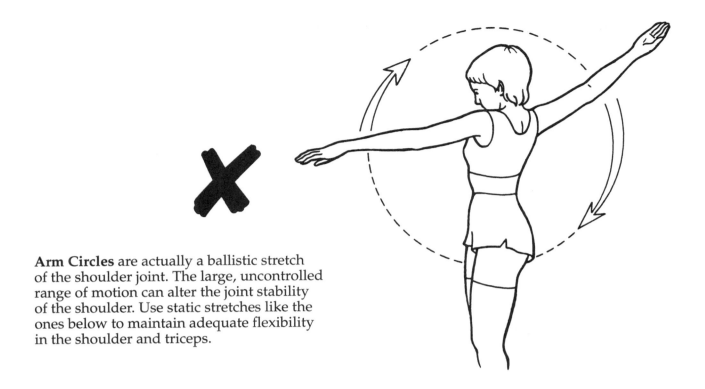

Arm Circles are actually a ballistic stretch of the shoulder joint. The large, uncontrolled range of motion can alter the joint stability of the shoulder. Use static stretches like the ones below to maintain adequate flexibility in the shoulder and triceps.

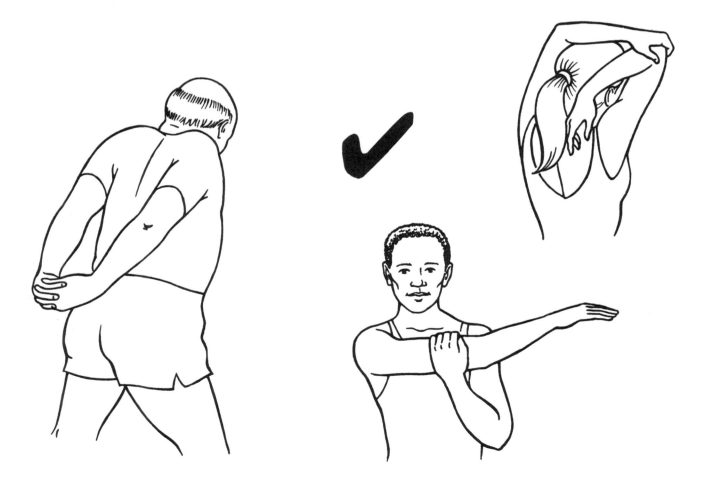

Stretching the Upper Body and Torso

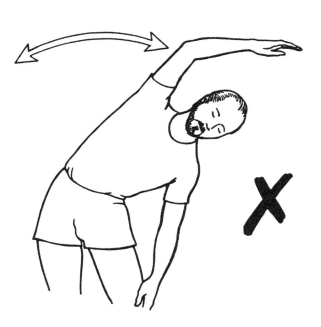

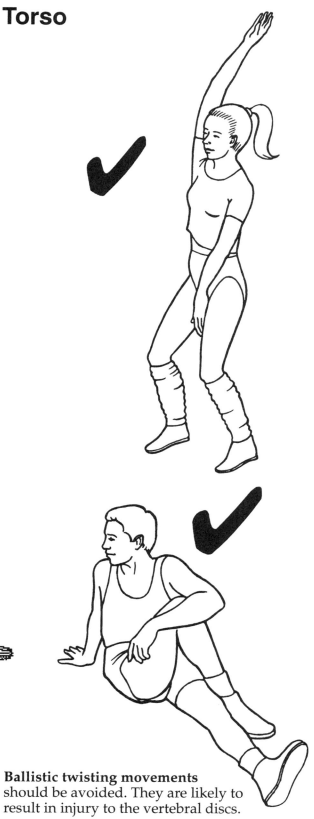

Sidebends should be limited to 20 degrees in order to prevent compression of the vertebral discs. They are not effective 'waist' exercises. You can stretch the same muscles by simply reaching in an upward direction with one arm. The knees should be bent to keep the spine in alignment.

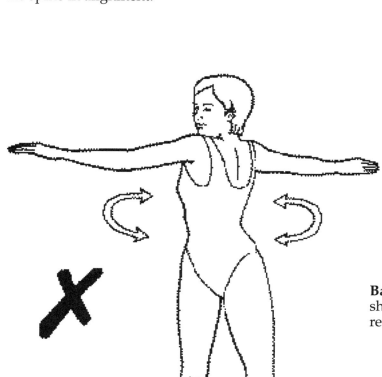

Ballistic twisting movements should be avoided. They are likely to result in injury to the vertebral discs.

Stretching the Abdominals

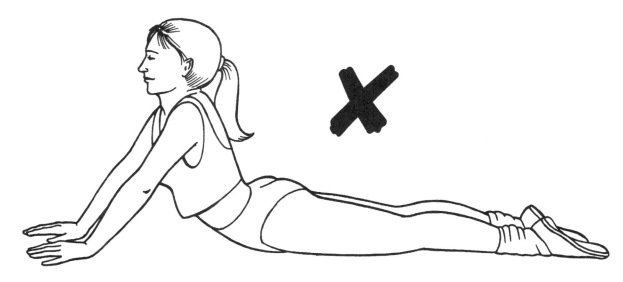

Never hyperextend the back to this degree-Arching the back while stretching or exercising is likely to cause injury due to compression of the spine and misalignment. It is good to lift the chest about six inches using the elbows for support.

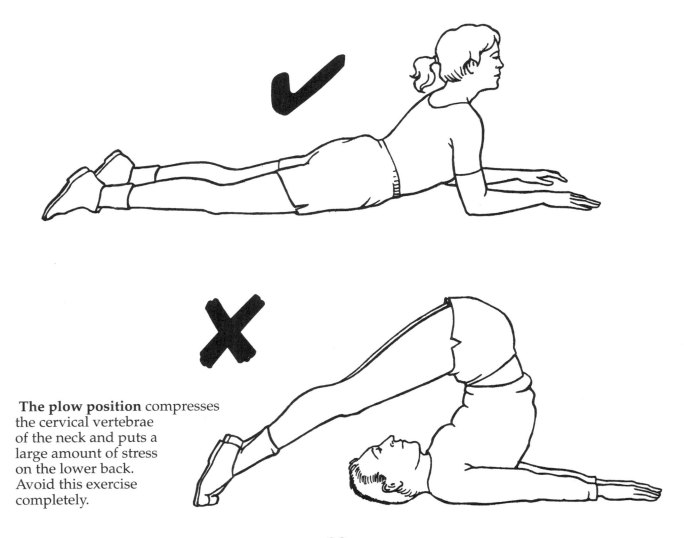

The plow position compresses the cervical vertebrae of the neck and puts a large amount of stress on the lower back. Avoid this exercise completely.

To safely stretch the lower back, pull your knees to your chest, hold beneath your knee caps (to prevent overbending of the knee joint), and curl up in a ball. Hold this position for at least 10 seconds.

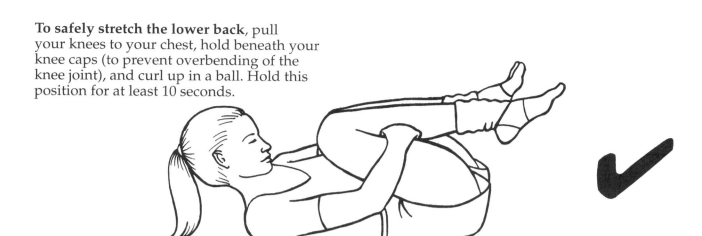

Another excellent stretch for the lower back involves lying on the back with one knee to the chest. Keep the other foot on the floor and press your lower back into the floor.

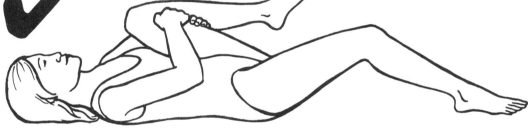

Stretching the Quadriceps

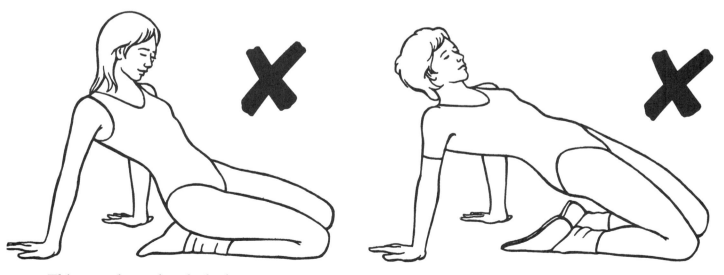

This stretch overbends the knee joint and places the back in a hyperextended position.

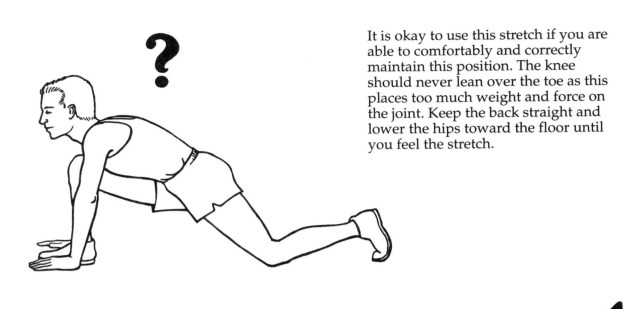

It is okay to use this stretch if you are able to comfortably and correctly maintain this position. The knee should never lean over the toe as this places too much weight and force on the joint. Keep the back straight and lower the hips toward the floor until you feel the stretch.

All three of these positions are safe if done correctly. Never pull on the foot. Press it into your hand and then squeeze your pelvis forward. You will feel a nice stretch in the quadricep but you should feel no pain in the hip or knee. Maintain the spine in a straight line at all times.

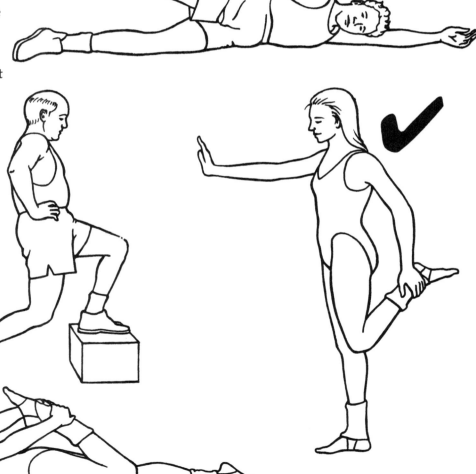

24

Stretching the Hamstrings

The stretches on this page involve extreme forward flexion of the spine and twisting and thus are contraindicated. Many are traditional positions that we have always done so it is difficult to remove them from your workout. Just remember that there are many safe and effective alternatives that could prevent lower back damage and other problems in the future.

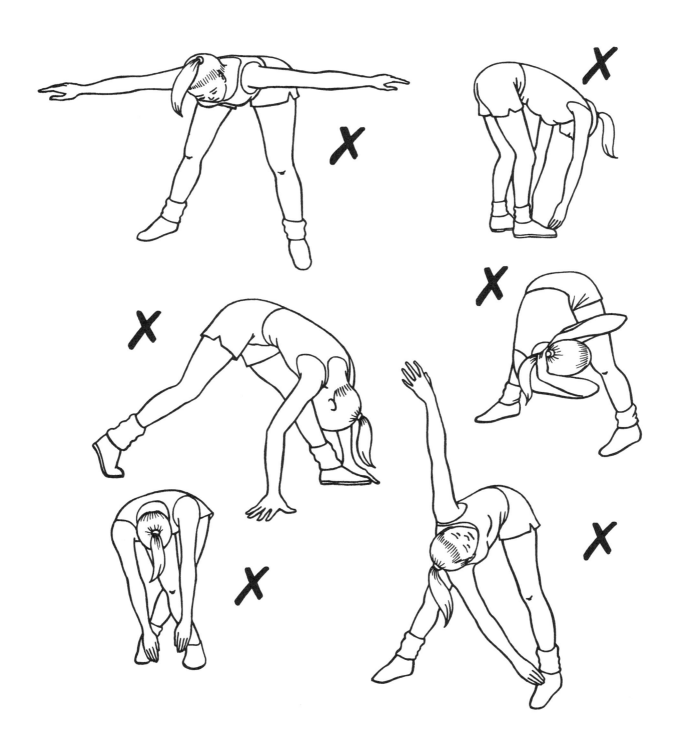

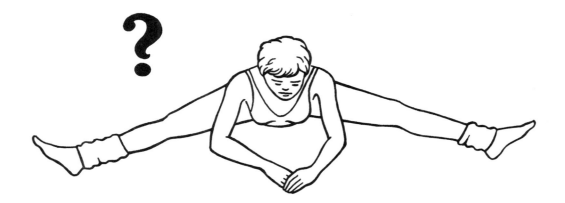

Sitting toe touches and straddle stretches are safe if and only if you are flexible enough to keep your spine in a straight line. There are more comfortable ways to stretch the hamstrings if this one causes you discomfort. If you prefer these positions, make sure you keep your knees soft and only go forward to the point of tension.

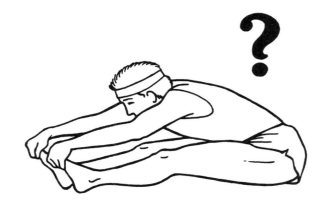

This hamstring and adductor stretch is contraindicated because bending to the side places the spine in a position of misalignment. Never bend more than 20 degrees to the side.

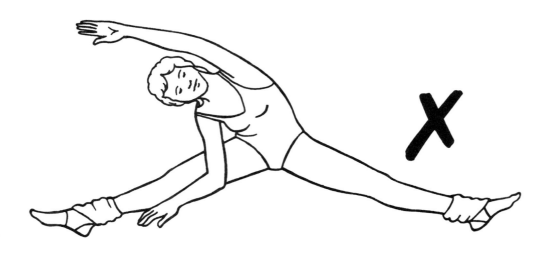

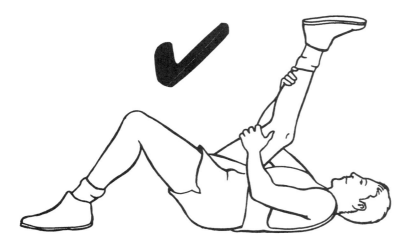

The safest way to increase flexibility in the hamstrings is on the back with one foot flat on the floor and the other knee pulled to your chest. Hold beneath your knee cap and slowly straighten your knee until you feel tension in the hamstring (never lock the knee). Hold for a minimum of 10 seconds.

It may be more convenient or comfortable to stand up to stretch. Just place your foot on a low step or bench, keep the knee bent, and bend from the hips until you feel the stretch on the back of your thigh.

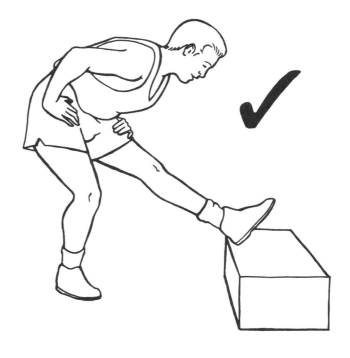

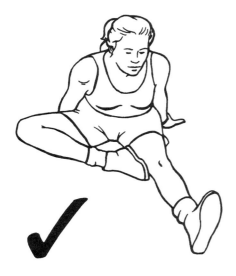

This modified position is much safer than the traditional 'hurdler's stretch' which places stress on the ligaments and tendons in the knee. When performing the modified hurdler keep the knee soft, the spine straight, and only go forward until you feel tension. If you feel the stretch sitting straight up, then hold that position.

Stretching the Adductors (Inner Thighs)

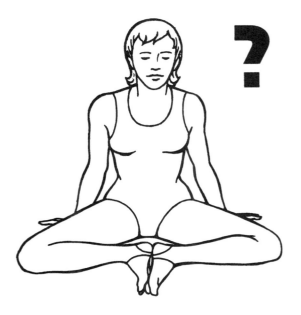

Safely stretch the adductors by sitting with the soles of the feet together and the arms supporting the back. Gently press the knees down and hold. Do not do this stretch if you have problems with your hips.

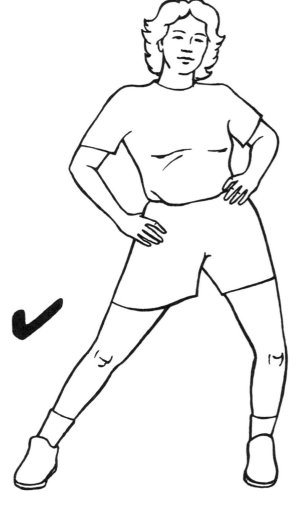

A modified hurdler position with the leg to the side will stretch the adductors also. Lean forward with your chest until you feel a mild stretch.

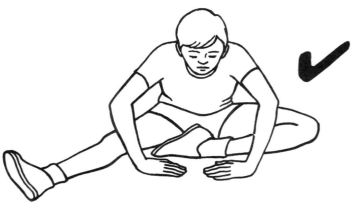

While standing you can lunge to one side and then tilt your hips to that same side. You will experience a mild stretch in the adductors of your straight leg.

Stretching the Gastrocnemius (Calf Muscle)

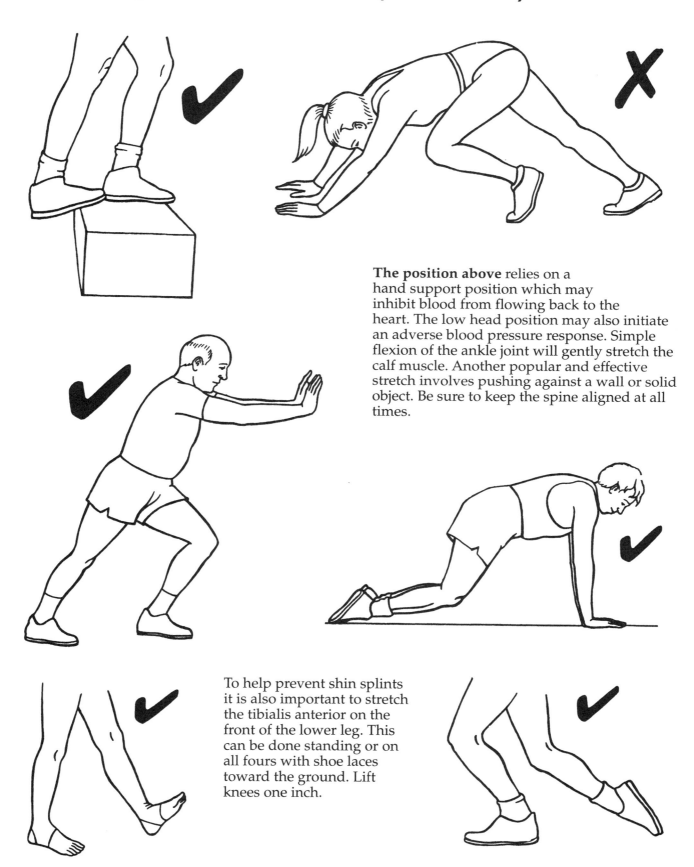

The position above relies on a hand support position which may inhibit blood from flowing back to the heart. The low head position may also initiate an adverse blood pressure response. Simple flexion of the ankle joint will gently stretch the calf muscle. Another popular and effective stretch involves pushing against a wall or solid object. Be sure to keep the spine aligned at all times.

To help prevent shin splints it is also important to stretch the tibialis anterior on the front of the lower leg. This can be done standing or on all fours with shoe laces toward the ground. Lift knees one inch.

Chapter Four

AEROBIC EXERCISE

Taking part in regular aerobic exercise will allow you to achieve cardiovascular health, help to control your weight, and will enhance physical and mental well-being. Although it is best to follow the guidelines of intensity, frequency, and duration outlined in this chapter, any amount of safe activity is better than nothing. So start moving!

Choosing an Aerobic Activity

There are many aerobic activities from which to choose. The decision should be based on your preferences, your present and past health and the equipment and facilities you have available to you. The activities below can all be considered aerobic. They are divided into low-impact and high-impact. Low-impact activities are not necessarily lower intensity. In fact, higher impact activities such as running and high level aerobic dance are associated with certain musculoskeletal injuries because of the vertical forces on the joints. One advantage of high-impact activity is that the weight-bearing exercise helps to maintain or increase bone mass. This may help prevent osteoporosis. There is plenty of evidence that lower impact exercises like walking and shallow water aerobics also maintain or build bone mass. If you choose a high-impact activity, make sure you have the proper shoes and a safe surface on which to exercise. It may be helpful to alternate low-impact with high-impact workouts. For example, running alternated with swimming. This is called 'cross-training' and helps to reduce boredom, increase fitness gains, and reduce the chance of injury. Cross training also promotes muscular balance and symmetry. People with health consideration such as knee or back problems should always choose low-impact exercises. Others simply find that low-impact is more enjoyable. Real life activities like taking out the trash or walking the dog can add up to significant health gains. Any activity in your day counts!

The key is moderation. You should be able to continue regular exercise for your entire life. Starting out with a fun, safe program and progressing gradually will increase your chances of sticking with an aerobic program.

Low-Impact Activities	**High-Impact Activities**
Walking/Hiking	Jogging
Aqua-Walking/Aqua-Jogging	Running
Swimming	High-Impact Aerobic Dance
Stationary Biking	Rope Skipping
Outdoor Cycling	
Low-Impact Aerobic Dance	**Real Life Activities**
Bench-Step Aerobics	Gardening
Aqua Aerobics	Mowing the Grass
Rowing	Playing with Young Children
Cross Country Skiing	Shopping the Mall
Stair Climbing	Vacuuming/Housework
Sliding	Change the Channel (without the remote)

This is not a complete list. Any activity which meets the requirements of frequency, duration, and intensity will achieve the desired results.

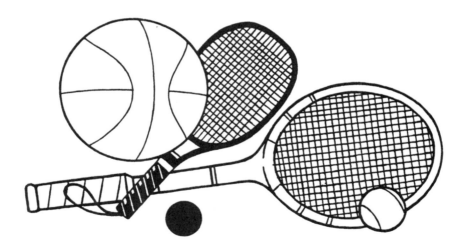

Sports such as tennis, racquetball, and basketball are sometimes considered aerobic, as long as there are not too many social or water breaks. They still burn calories, reduce stress, and provide varying amounts of aerobic benefit.

Frequency, Duration, and Intensity of Aerobic Exercise

Based on Guidelines from the American College of Sports Medicine

Frequency

Research has demonstrated that significant gains in cardiovascular endurance can result with a minimum of three non-consecutive days of aerobic exercise per week. Unless you wish to train for a marathon or other athletic event, three days a week is plenty to improve your health and fitness. If weight control or weight loss is a priority, however, exercising aerobically four to seven days a week will burn more calories. In this case extreme caution is necessary in order to avoid overuse injuries. For sedentary individuals and those with health problems, even short bursts of activity each day lead to health benefits. For example, 10 minutes of walking. Your total activity should add up to 30 minutes of moderate–intensity exercise on most days of the week.

Duration

To achieve gains in cardiovascular endurance it is necessary to raise the heart rate into a level where you feel moderately exerted. 30 or more minutes are recommended, however, the longer you exercise the greater the chance of injury. Progression is very important so start with 5 or 10 minutes and add a few minutes with each workout until you reach your goal. Even if you only have time for 10 or 15 minutes this is better than skipping your workout. One study demonstrated greater weight loss for those doing 10 minutes 4 times per day over those doing 40 consecutive minutes. In other words, we're not sure it has to be consecutive. Any activity added to your day will be beneficial.

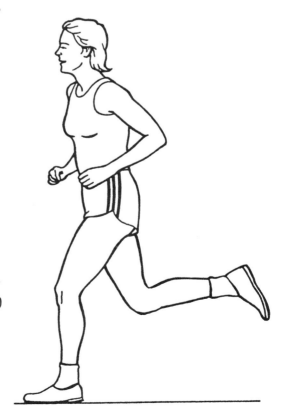

Always finish your aerobic activity with at least 5 minutes of walking or low-level activity. If you stand still while your heart rate is elevated, the blood will pool in your legs and you may become faint or dizzy. Keep moving so the muscles can pump blood back to your heart. When your heart rate falls below 120 beats/minute (100 beats/minute if you are over 50) it is usually safe to stop.

Jogging is a popular aerobic activity.

33

Intensity

Research has shown that in order for cardiovascular training effects to occur, one has to overload the cardiovascular system a minimal amount during aerobic exercise to achieve increased endurance and efficiency. When you exercise, your heart beats faster to meet the demands of your muscles for more blood and oxygen. This is the most difficult component to monitor accurately. It is also important to monitor intensity on the high end. If you push too hard you may be working at an intensity so high that your *aerobic* (with oxygen) energy system cannot meet the body's demand for oxygen. At this point your *anaerobic* (without oxygen) system begins to produce much of the energy used. Both aerobic and anaerobic exercise burn calories and increase endurance. Deconditioned individuals are better off working at a lower intensity for a longer duration or in several sessions with rest in between. Also, for high risk participants it can be dangerous to exercise at a very high intensity. The intensity of an aerobic exercise session can be monitored in several ways. The best method is a combination of Target Heart Zone and Perceived Exertion.

Perceived Exertion

The 'Perceived Exertion' method relies on you to feel how hard you are working using cues such as rate of breathing and ability to talk in a normal voice. The simplest form of this is called the 'Talk Test.' If you can sing (very little exertion) you are not working your cardiovascular system hard enough; if you can't say a normal sentence (gasping) you are pushing too hard. Many people use a very useful system called the Borg RPE Scale. You rate (with a verbal description) the physical strain you are experiencing during exercise. Stay between 4 (Somewhat Strong) and 6 (Strong) for a safe and effective cardiovascular workout.

Borg RPE Scale

0	Nothing at All
0.5	Very, very weak
1	Very weak
2	Weak
3	Moderate
4	Somewhat strong
5	Strong
6	
7	Very Strong
8	
9	
10	Very, very strong
*	Maximal

Stay in This Zone (4, 5, 6)

The proper heart rate range is called the 'Target Heart Zone' and is based on your maximal heart rate. It is best to have a Graded Exercise Test to determine your exact maximal heart rate. This is not practical for most individuals. Estimating is the next best choice. The Karvonen Method and Age-Based Target Heart Zone are described below. They are best used in combination with Perceived Exertion measurements.

The intensity level should be based on factors such as previous exercise experience and current fitness level. For most healthy people, a range somewhere between 40% and 85% of their maximal heart rate is best. If you have never exercised before, you should start with a lower intensity level and progress gradually.

Some medications for high blood pressure and other problems increase or decrease the heart rate. In this case intensity cannot be measured by monitoring the heart rate and a physician and exercise physiologist should be consulted to determine the correct mode and level of exercise.

The best method is a combination of Perceived Exertion and Target Heart Zone. Since, your heart rate during exercise is related to how you feel, after a while you will be able to tell when you are working at the correct intensity without checking your pulse so often. A chest strap heart rate monitor is very accurate and effective.

Monitoring Your Pulse

Heart rate is a relatively accurate means of monitoring exercise intensity. Heart rates should be taken several times during the aerobic segment of your workout and once afterward to monitor cool-down. When you first begin an exercise program it may be advantageous to take it more often or to use a pulse monitor. Take your pulse either on the thumbside of your wrist (radial pulse) or the groove in your neck (carotid pulse). Make sure you use your first two fingers and not your thumb. Your thumb has its own pulse and may cause you to count inaccurately. Never press too hard. Count for 6 seconds and multiply by 10 or simply add a zero. For example, if your pulse beats 15 times in 6 seconds, your heart rate is 150. It may take a while for you to become proficient. It helps to practice taking your pulse so you can do it quickly and accurately when exercising.

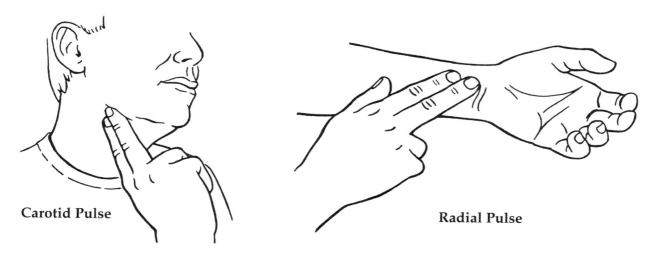

Carotid Pulse   **Radial Pulse**

Determining Your Resting Pulse Rate

Immediately after awakening from a good night's sleep lie very still and find your pulse. Do not sit up or stand up. Count it for a full minute. This is your resting pulse rate. Use it in the equation below to calculate your Target Heart Zone. If you have not been exercising regularly you can expect your resting heart rate to decrease as you become more fit. This means your heart will pump more oxygenated blood to your body with fewer beats.

Determining Your Maximal Heart Rate

Choice 1:   Number is based on an actual max exercise test _____beats/minute

Choice 2:   220—Age = _____beats/minute (low estimate/beginners)

Choice 3:   210—(0.5 x age) = _____beats/minute (high estimate/more fit)

Calculating Your Target Heart Zone

Follow the Karvonen equation to determine your individual target zone. If you are on medications that lower or raise heart rate (i.e. beta blockers) you cannot use heart rate as an accurate measure of intensity. Consult with your physician and exercise professional.

The Karvonen Formula

1.   Subtract your resting HR from your maximal HR to obtain your HR reserve

(_____) − (_____) = _____Heart Rate Reserve
Maximal HR   Resting HR

2.   Then, calculate 60 percent and 80 percent of your HR reserve and add each value to your resting HR to obtain your THZ range.

(_____) × 0.60 = (_____) + (_____) = _____
HR Reserve Intensity   RHR   Low Target HR

(_____) × 0.80 = (_____) + (_____) = _____
HR Reserve Intensity   RHR   High Target HR

Example

A 45 year old female wants to determine her Target Heart Zone. She takes her pulse upon awakening and finds it to be 69 beats per minute.

1. 220 − 45 (age) = 175 (Low Estimated Maximal Heart Rate)
   or 210 − 45(0.5)= 187.55 (High Estimated Maximal Heart Rate)
   She is a beginner so she chooses the low estimate

2. 175 (MHR) − 69 (Resting HR) = 106 (Heart Rate Reserve)

3. 106 (HRR) × 0.60 (Intensity) = 63.6 +69 (RHR) = 132.6 (Target HR)
   106 (HRR) × 0.80 (Intensity) = 84.8 +69 (RHR) = 153.8 (Target HR)

4. Round Numbers up or down   **130** (Lower End of Target Zone)
   155 (Higher End of Target Zone)

She should maintain a pulse of *130 to 155* throughout her 20-60 minutes of aerobic exercise (13 to 16 beats in six seconds).

The Bell Curve Concept

Use the 'bell curve' technique for designing your aerobic workout. Start out slowly (at the bottom of your THZ). Slowly increase the intensity and keep your heart rate near the top of your THZ for 10 to 15 minutes. Taper down at the end so when you complete a total of 20 to 40 minutes you are back down to the lower level of your target zone. Always finish with a low-intensity cool-down to bring your heart rate below 120 beats/minute (100 beats/min for those 50 or older)

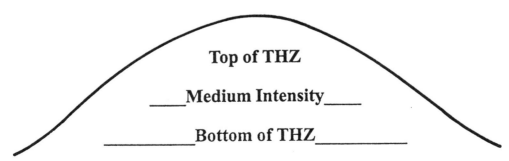

Top of THZ

____Medium Intensity____

_____Bottom of THZ_____

Total Aerobic Workout should last at least 20 minutes!

Interval Training

As you achieve cardiovascular fitness you can vary your workout by alternating high and low intensity during your aerobic phase. Intervals involve working a little harder than 'steady rate' or what is physically comfortable. This acceleration in level of effort is followed by a moderate recovery interval or time period, when activity returns to an easily sustainable level of effort. Intervals mimic the ups and downs of everyday life. Research shows interval training can build extra stamina (endurance), increase fat loss and calorie burning, and improve personal performance. For example, work at the highest level of your THZ for 1 minute, then slow down to the lowest intensity of your THZ for 2-3 minutes. Repeat several cycles. You can do a longer work interval as your endurance improves. Try doing one interval workout each week along with your steady state or bell curve workout. This method has been shown to give added edurance benefits by challenging the cardiovascular system.

Another Option: ACSM/CDC Exercise Lite!

Vigorous activity has been associated with increased longevity and many health benefits, however, some people are not motivated to stick with strict exercise guidelines. Studies show that many inactive people dislike vigorous exercise. There is also less risk of cardiac and other injuries with less intensity. Many sedentary people and others with health problems would benefit from moderate intensity activity. The American College of Sports Medicine and the Centers for Disease Control and Prevention have made recommendations for this group. Performing activity based on the guidelines in this chapter will give you the most benefit, but fitness is a continuum. The idea is to do more than you've been doing. Any progress will improve your health and may lead to more activity in the future.

They recommend 'to accumulate 30 minutes or more of moderate-intensity physical activity on most, preferably all, days of the week.' Short bouts of 8 to 10 minutes several times per day. Activities such as a brisk walk or mowing the lawn would qualify. Another way to keep track is to burn around 200 Calories per day doing moderate activity or 1,000 to 1,400 in any given seven day period. The important idea is consistency. This plan will start you on the road to better fitness.

Safety Tips for Common Aerobic Activities

Walking

Many people are choosing a walking program to achieve aerobic benefits. The advantages are numerous. You can walk anywhere, it costs very little money and you can continue for a lifetime of safe exercise. Sometimes it is difficult to bring the heart rate into the target zone but this can be facilitated with light hand weights (do not grip too tightly). Arms should pump front to back, bent at a right angle. Do not twist your torso as you stride. Ankle weights are discouraged because they increase the force of impact on the feet and joints. Proper shoes are also imperative to prevent injury.

Jogging

Jogging is an important part of the lifestyle of literally millions of people. It is an effective way to increase fitness and health. It requires very little equipment and you can do it almost anywhere. Proper shoes are a must. If you are a new jogger go to a reputable dealer who can help you choose a running shoe to serve your individual needs. Replace your shoes as soon as they wear out to guard against stress injuries.

There is no one correct way to jog but some simple guidelines may prevent an injury. Stand erect and keep the spine as straight as possible. Your arms should be relaxed and bent at the elbow. They should swing front to back with no side to side motion. The most important factor is the way your foot makes contact with the running surface. Land on the back third of your foot, roll forward and lift from the front of your foot to push forward for the next step. The running surface is also a potential source of chronic injury. Smooth, even surfaces are best. Cement and concrete are very hard and thus result in more injuries than grass or track surfaces.

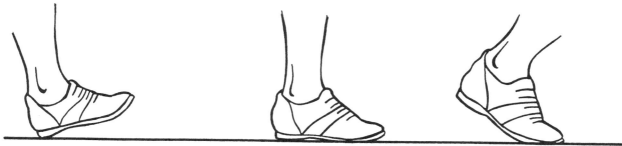

The proper foot strike sequence when running or jogging.

Aerobic Dance

The crucial ingredient for a safe and effective class is a trained and concerned instructor. Check qualifications and background before you begin the class. Other important features include a proper surface such as a wooden floor or a specially designed aerobic floor, a controlled environment that is not too hot or too cold and appropriate, well-fitting footwear. Recent studies indicate that the arm movements in aerobic dance may produce a higher heart rate than other activities even though the intensity (oxygen consumption) is the same. To achieve maximal benefit use more lower body movements like lunges, knee lifts and kicks. Try to travel more and avoid too much repetition. Avoid instructors that include any twists, extreme sidebends, or forward flexion or who do not include a thermal warm-up and final stretching.

Swimming

This activity is perfect for almost everyone, but especially those with orthopedic problems, joint discomfort, pregnant women, the elderly, obese or overweight individuals, and many others. The water supports the weight of your body so there are few overuse or impact problems. To assure your safety make sure you are comfortable in the water and that there are lifeguards available at all times. Cleanliness and proper maintenance of the pool facility are also important.

Aqua-Aerobics/Water Walking

Exercising in the water does not have to involve swimming. Many athletes train in the water to avoid excessive impact on their joints while still maintaining a very high intensity level. Water exercise can take many forms including water walking or jogging in shallow water, deep water jogging, aqua-aerobics, bench stepping in the water, interval training, circuit training, and more. New studies indicate that swimming may not be helpful in building bone density but that aqua-aerobics, walking, and jogging in shallow water is beneficial (feet landing on bottom of pool).

Bench Step Aerobics

Bench Stepping is extremely effective and safe if done correctly. The intensity can be the same as running but the impact is similar to walking. This means you can get a very hard workout in a short amount of time. Safety is a primary concern. The instructor must be specially trained to cue and instruct properly. Some people with pre-existing knee problems may find that this activity aggravates their injury. Wait until you are completely healed and begin slowly. Other concerns and tips include:

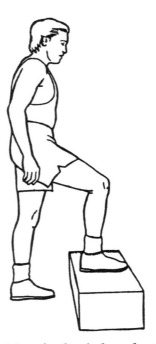

The proper position for basic bench stepping.

1) Make sure your stepping surface is not too high, start with 4 inches and gradually progress. Very few people have long enough legs to use a step higher than 10 inches. 2) Place your whole foot on the bench with every move. 3) Use music that is the appropriate speed (120 to 126 beats/min). 4) Step down close to the bench so you will effectively use gravity. 5) Extend all the way every time you step up on the bench but do not lock your knee. 6) Never step forward off the bench 7) Jumping onto the bench (power moves) are recommended only for advanced steppers. Jumping off the bench onto the floor is never recommended.

Stair Steppers

This is a vigorous exercise since you have to raise your body against gravity while stepping forward. Make sure you get instruction on each individual machine. Gripping the handrails means less intensity than letting go. You can adjust step height and step rate to arrive at the appropriate level.

Cycling or Spinning

Progress slowly, walking and other aerobic activities will not prepare your leg and thigh muscles for intense cycling. If cycling along roads, wear appropriate safety equipment (i.e. helmet and reflective materials) and observe proper rules and regulations of the road. Stationary biking is great for winter months and rainy days, however, do not invest in expensive equipment until you have proven you will stick with it. Walk for several months and then reward yourself with a stationary cycle. Spinning is fun and very high intensity. You have the benefit of an instructor for safty and motivation.

Cross-Training

You can achieve a greater cardiovascular endurance level by varying your aerobic activities. This helps prevent boredom and decreases overuse injuries. Studies have also shown more effective weight and fat loss and better muscular balance in people who cross train. For example, walking Monday, Wednesday, and Friday and cycling on Tuesday and Thursday.

Chapter Five

MUSCULAR STRENGTH AND ENDURANCE

This portion of the workout can last anywhere from ten to sixty minutes depending on the time, space, and equipment available. It normally follows the aerobic section but can be done on alternate days or immediately after the warm-up.

The Concept of Overload

If a muscle, muscle group, or the cardiovascular system is worked harder than it is normally accustomed, it will eventually improve and become more efficient. As one level becomes less demanding you can work slightly harder the next time and you will continue to improve. This concept applies to aerobic exercise as well as to weight training and calisthenics.

The Spot Reducing Myth

Body fat cannot be altered by specific spot reduction exercises. When you exercise, you utilize energy produced by metabolizing fat from all of the regions of your body, not just the muscles involved in that specific exercise. Calisthenics and weight training exercises work to build and tone muscle but burn very little fat. Body fat is a primary energy source only when exercising aerobically within your target heart zone. The amount of fat burned will depend on the duration and intensity of your workout. It is also a myth that muscles will turn to fat if you cease exercising. They are two distinct types of tissue.

If you are trying to control your weight by decreasing your caloric and fat intake you must exercise to maintain lean body mass. Otherwise you will lose muscle and fat. Aerobic activity is not enough to accomplish this goal. You must include strength training. The long term benefit of weight training and body sculpting is increased muscle mass. Because muscle is more active metabolically than fat, even at rest, you will burn more calories all the time. This is one of the key ways that a complete fitness program, including strength training, will help you control your weight.

Muscular Strength Development

The key to significant strength increases is the amount of tension produced by a muscle. The way to improve muscular strength is to perform exercises that require few repetitions but involve large amounts of tension. The best method of accomplishing significant strength gains is through resistance training. Strength training is crucial for back health and prevention of injury to the joints. Weight training for strength will produce significant hypertrophy (increased muscle size) in the male because of the hormone testosterone. Females need not worry about becoming muscle bound since they do not have high levels of testosterone.

Significant strength gains can also be achieved by adding resistance to regular exercises. For example, abdominal curls with weights in the hands or upper body work with rubberized bands as shown in this chapter. It is now agreed that including a muscular strength component is important for all people. Consult your physician prior to lifting weights or using bands if you have high blood pressure, are pregnant, have Carpal Tunnel Syndrome, or any other injury or condition that could limit physical activity.

Muscular Endurance Development

By overloading the muscles so that their need for oxygen is increased, the ability to continue sustained and repeated contractions is enhanced. This is accomplished by working the muscles frequently and by using high numbers of repetitions. Weight training and rubberized bands as well as numerous calisthenic exercises will increase muscular endurance.

A combination of strength training and endurance training is optimal for achieving benefits related to health. Increased strength in the appropriate muscle groups will help correct muscle imbalances, preventing back pain, knee injuries and other problems. Increased endurance will result in better muscle tone and an improved ability to carry out daily tasks.

Alternatives for Building Strength and Endurance

Calisthenics: Abdominal curl-ups, modified and regular push-ups, leg lifts, tricep lifts, etc. require no special equipment and can greatly enhance muscular conditioning. Mats or a carpeted area are necessary for proper cushioning. In an outdoor area a towel can be placed on the grass.

Weight Training: If weight training equipment is available the program outlined in this chapter should be used to increase overall strength, endurance, and muscle balance: Since there is a large variety of equipment, make sure you are oriented and instructed as to proper use of the equipment and proper technique.

Rubberized Resistance: Many people do not have convenient access to weight training equipment or facilities. Studies have demonstrated that adding resistance to our muscle work greatly enhances muscular strength. Exercising with rubberized resistance such as the 6-Foot Challenge Bands® and Lower Body Challenge Bands® shown in this chapter is a quick, convenient way to build muscular strength and endurance at home, at work, on vacation, or anywhere. There are several brands of rubber bands that can be used to increase strength and endurance. Some, like the CHALLENGE® bands come in different levels of resistance. See Resource Guide to order CHALLENGE® bands.

The following prescription should be used to increase overall strength, endurance and muscle balance: The American College of Sports Medicine recommends at least two non-consecutive days per week, although three days would allow faster progress.

1 or 3 Sets with weights or bands - Studies indicate that one set is as good as 2 but 3 gives you slightly better results. For fitness purposes this is good news. Busy people can achieve almost all the benefits with just one set. The key is to be warm before you start and to use moderate to heavy workloads.

Proper Progression 8 to 12 Repetitions - Begin at 8 repetitions, work up to 12. This gives you the best mix of strength and endurance. When 12 is easy, increase the weight slightly and go back to 8 repetitions. This way you will continue to increase strength and endurance.

Light to moderate weight or resistance - Choose a weight such that you feel the fatigue on the last 3-4 repetitions.

Proper Body Position - If any position or exercise causes discomfort it should be discontinued immediately. The back and the knee are most vulnerable to injury so avoid locking the knee and never hyperextend (arch) the lower back while lifting weights.

Vary Your Workout - Every few months, change your workout slightly so you will continue to improve (type of exercise, speed of contraction, etc).

Slower is Better - New studies are showing that you will see greater increases in strength if you go very slow through the whole contraction. This is difficult to do because you are not able to utilize momentum. You may need to decrease your weight in order to slow down. Ten seconds on the positive contraction and four seconds on the negative (lowering) contraction.

For Muscle Balance: If your time is limited, do these first.
Abdominals
Hamstrings
Rhomboids (Upper Back)
Erector Spinae (Lower Back)
Triceps
Rotator Cuff
Abductors (Outer Thighs)
Deltoids

For Additional Toning and Strengthening:
Pectorals (Chest)
Biceps
Adductors (Inner Thighs)
Gastrocnemius (Calves)
Quadriceps
Hip Flexors

Safety Tips for Weight Training and Muscle Work

- Never perform muscle work without completing a circulatory/thermal warm-up.

- When performing standing exercises simply bend your knees. This is called the 'neutral pelvic position' and puts your spine in the best position to support weight and movement.

- Never lock the knees or elbows during any exercise. Maintain enough control so that you straighten the joint without locking or snapping.

- The highest priority should be to avoid hyperextending the neck, the back, or the knees. Keep your spine in alignment at all times.

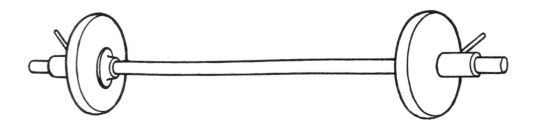

- Deep knee bends or squats should be avoided. They place too much stress on the knees and back.

- Avoid exercises which involve forward flexion of the spine (for example, bent over rows).

Working the Upper Body

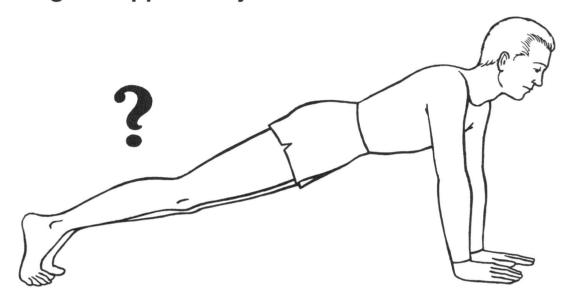

When performing push-ups make sure you are strong enough to keep your spine in line. The back should not arch and the buttocks should not raise to dip the chin. When you approach the 'up' position do not snap your elbows into a locked position. Modified push-ups do not require as much strength as regular push-ups and allow better control of body position.

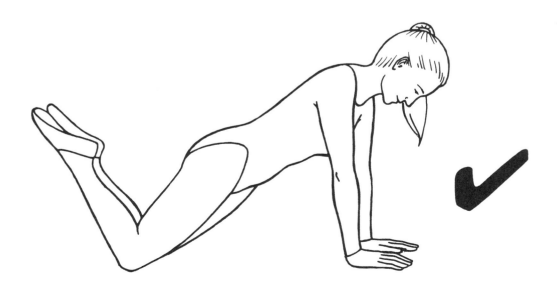

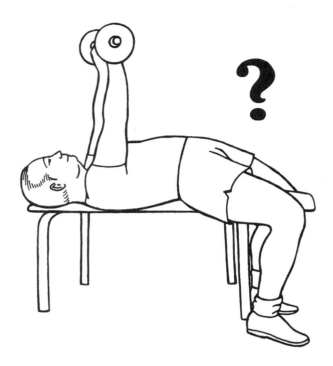

Avoid arching the back while performing any weight training exercise on a bench. Putting your feet on the bench with the knees bent will protect your lower back. Also remember to control each movement so that you never snap or lock a joint.

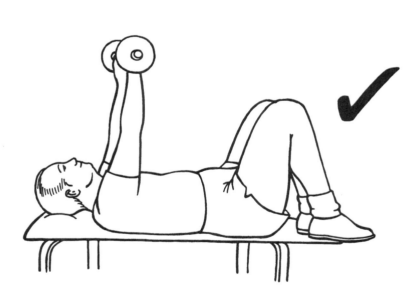

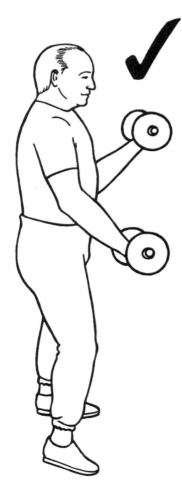

When lifting weights in a standing position, keep the knees bent. Each movement should follow the full range of motion for that particular joint.

Exercising With Rubberized Resistance

Safety Tips:

Bend your knees on all exercises.

Do not hyperextend or lock your joints.

Never hold your breath. Exhale on the hardest exertion.

Control every movement. No bouncing or jerking.

There are limitless exercises that can be performed with the 6-FOOT CHALLENGE BAND® AND THE LOWER BODY CHALLENGE BAND®. Here is a complete routine that you can do in ten-fifteen minutes to get a well-rounded upper and lower body workout. A video is available if you need help following the exercise. See the Resource Guide in the appendices.

Pectorals/Chest

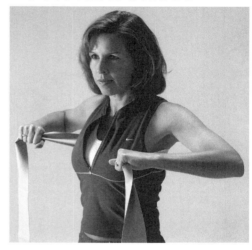

Starting Position Wrap band behind your back. Grab each side close to your underarms. Bend knees.

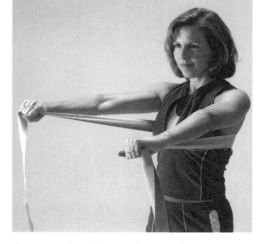

Contraction Extend straight out. Exhale as you extend. Inhale as you return to the starting position.

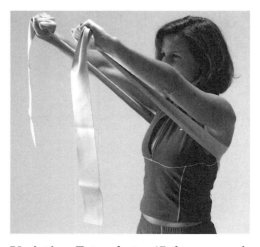

Variation Extend at a 45 degree angle.

Upper Back/Chest

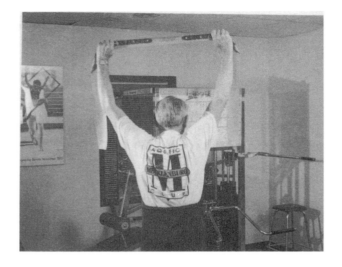

Starting Position Hold band above your head with hands about eight inches apart. Bend knees. Tuck pelvis under.

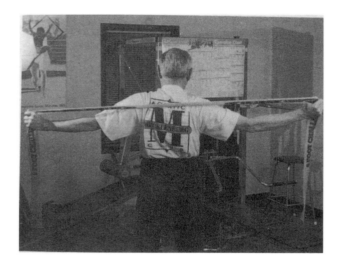

ContractionPull out and down behind your head, bringing shoulder blades together. Do not arch the lower back. Return to the starting position. If this position causes any discomfort, pull down to the front only.

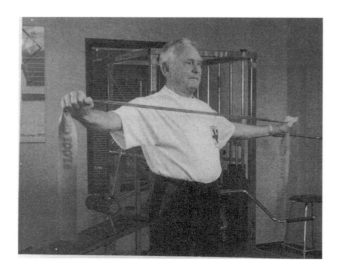

Variation Pull out and down to the front. Return to the starting position.

Biceps

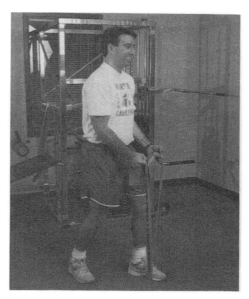

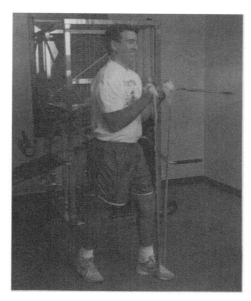

Starting Position Bend knees. Place center of band under one foot and grab each end. Hold as if you were holding candles straight up. This will keep your wrists from bending.

Contraction Slowly curl. The only motion is from the elbow down. Lower very slowly to the starting position and repeat.

Deltoids

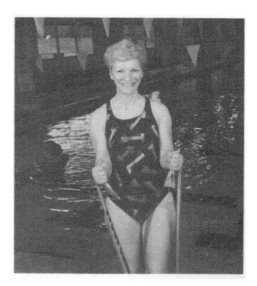

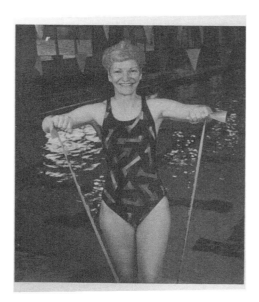

Starting Position Bend knees. Place center of band under one foot. Grab band and wrap over the top of each hand.

Contraction Lift arms as a unit, leading with the elbows. Do not lift higher than shoulder level.

Triceps

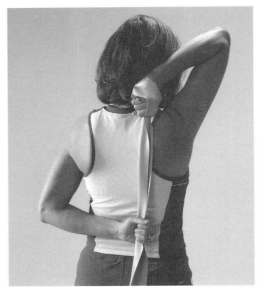

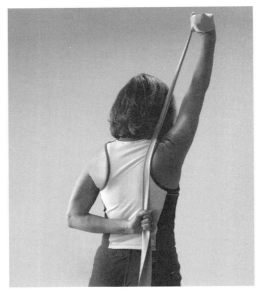

Starting Position Bend knees. Hold band in your right hand with your arm by your ear.
Stabilization Bend elbow and grab with the left hand behind the back.

Contraction Stabilize the left hand and slowly extend the right arm. Repeat on the other side.

Triceps (alternative)

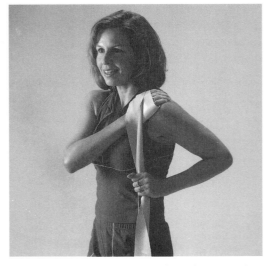

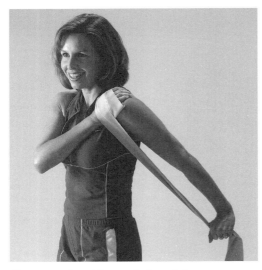

Starting Position Wrap band around your left hand and place on the right shoulder. Grab with the right hand.

Contraction Extend the right arm down along your side. Repeat on the other side.

Rotator Cuff

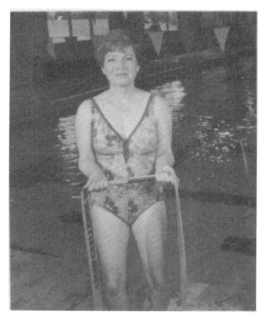 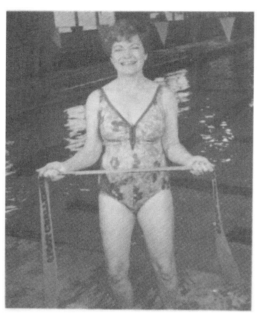

Starting Position Hold band close together, palms up, with elbows glued to your waist.

Contraction Pull straight out to the side 4-8 inches. Slowly return to starting position.

Shoulder Shrugs

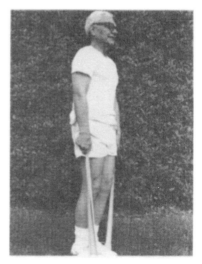 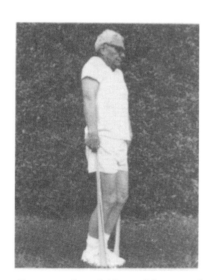

Starting Position Stand on center of band with both feet. Grab each end.Bend knees

Contraction Lift and lower the shoulders. Also try forward and backward shoulder rolls.

Lower Body Challenge

The following exercises are designed as an extremely effective lower body strengthening and sculpting program that can be completed in 5-10 minutes. All exercises are performed with a looped, latex band (Lower Body Challenge Band®) that is long enough to allow for full range of motion. Repeat each movement 8 times. Pay careful attention to safety instructions to avoid any stress on the knee.

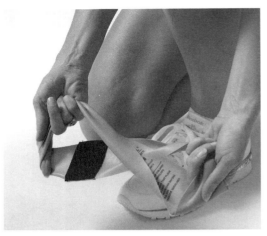

Starting Position: Twist the band into a figure eight.

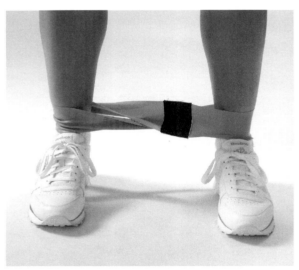

Place one foot in each loop so band is around ankles. Socks keep the band from rolling. This is the starting position for all four exercises.

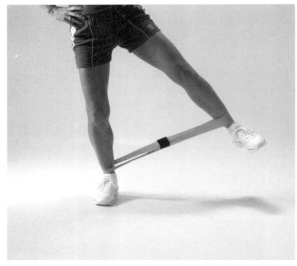

Abductor Exercise (Outer Thigh): Keeping knees bent during the entire exercise, lift leg 45 degrees to the side. Keep knee pointed to the front. Hold onto a chair or rail for balance if needed.

Hamstrings and Gluteals

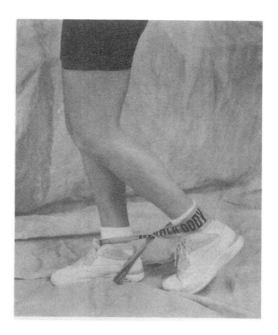

Starting Position: Start with figure 8 around ankles. Slide one loop under your right heel. Knees are squeezed together.

Hamstring Curls: Keeping knees together, lift left leg to a 90 degree angle. Slowly return to starting position. Repeat 8 times. Then pulse 8 times at the top of the contraction (isometric contraction). Repeat on the other side.

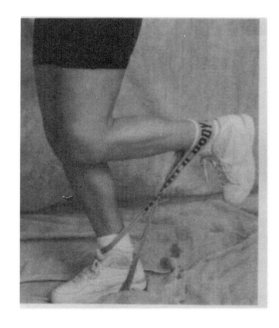

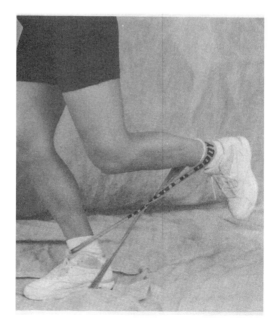

Gluteals: Curl up to 90 degrees. Then with foot flexed, push your heel straight back about four inches. Return to 90 degree position. Repeat 8 times.

Quadriceps

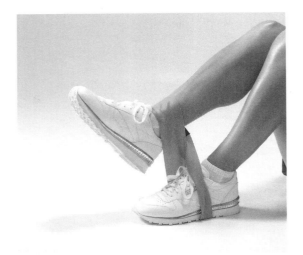

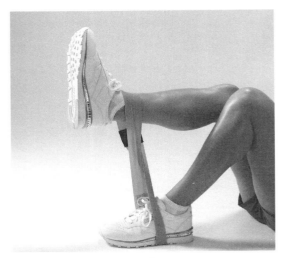

Starting Position: Sit down and place hands on the floor behind you for support. Start with figure 8 around ankles. Slide one loop under your right heel. The other loop is around your sock. Knees are squeezed together.

Contraction: Extend your lower leg about 15 degrees until it is almost straight but not locked. Return to position where band is almost slack. Repeat 8 times. Then extend, hold and point your toe, then flex and return to starting position. Finally pulse 8 times at the top of the contraction.

Adductors (Inner Thighs)

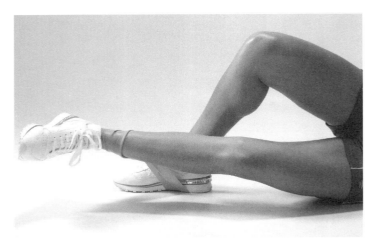

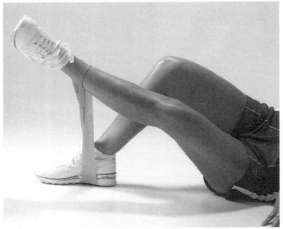

Starting Position: Lie on your side with figure 8 around ankles. Keep your back straight and slide one loop under your back heel. You must keep your front knee bent at all times.

Contraction: Slowly lift your front leg as a unit. Use your inner thigh to lift, not your ankle. Repeat 8 times. Pulse at the top 8 times.

Working the Abdominals

The abdominals include the rectus abdominus, the transverse abdominus and the internal and external obliques. It is important to strengthen all of these core support muscles. Traditionally, full sit-ups, elbow to knee positions, and straight leg lifts have been the preferred exercises for strengthening the abdominals. The problem is that these exercises actually contract the hip flexors (iliopsoas) which are already strong. This cheats the weaker abdominal group and increases the degree of muscle imbalance. Once you curl your torso past about 30 degrees, the hip flexors take over. This is why you feel your legs tighten as you do a full sit-up. To prevent this problem, pull your heels as close to your body as possible or cross your legs straight in the air. You will not be able to come up as far but now you are isolating your abdominals and making them do all the work.

Recent research tells us that we need to perform fewer repetitions when working the abdominals and add more resistance. The strength gained from this method is much more beneficial in providing muscular support for the spine and preventing other imbalance problems. In other words, quality is much more important than quantity. The side benefit is less time spent working the abdominals. You can use bands, weights, or gravity to achieve this additional resistance.

Go slowly and control each curl-up. Exhale as you curl up (on the exertion) and inhale as you lower. Come up as far as you can without tightening your thighs, then return completely to the starting position. This will insure that you increase abdominal strength through the full range of movement. A simple test to check your form: Place your hand on your abdominals with your thumb on the lowest rib and your pinky on your hip bone. Concentrate on bringing these two points closer together every time you curl up.

Avoid full sit-ups. Support your neck if needed. Do not pull forward on your head. When you become fatigued it is tempting to pull on your head in order to complete the sit-up. This may result in cervical vertebrae damage. If you feel the contraction in your hips you are coming up too far or improperly. The straight-leg position places great strain on the lower back. By placing your feet under a bar you are allowing the hip flexors to do even more of the work.

Avoid elbow to knee exercises. They primarily work the hip flexors and place strain on the neck and spine. The 'six inches off the floor' exercise is extremely dangerous. It places tremendous strain on the lower back and depends almost totally on the hip flexors.

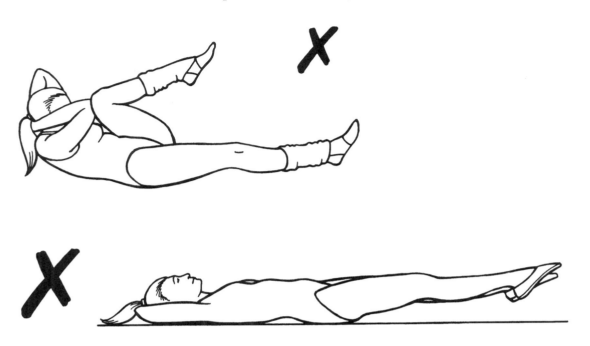

The basic curl up is safe and effective. Heels should be about 6 inches from the buttocks. Back is relaxed (neutral position) and may have a slight space between the floor and lower back. Curl up, bringing rib cage closer to pelvis. To achieve a bigger contraction perform a pelvic tilt as you curl up. Always return completely to the neutral starting position. Arms can be crossed on the chest, touching the ear lobes or shoulders, or supporting the neck. You can also perform chest presses, bicep curls, or other arm motions as you curl up. To work the obliques (side abdominal muscles), tilt knees slightly to the side and perform the same curl-up with a pelvic tilt. Change the type of contraction often: single lift and lower, slow lift, hold and lower, pulse at the top, up quickly, slowly lower. This will challenge the abdominals and allow them to fatigue more quickly. Using a stability ball is an excellent way to work the abdominals. You get a larger range of motion and more involvement of all muscle groups.

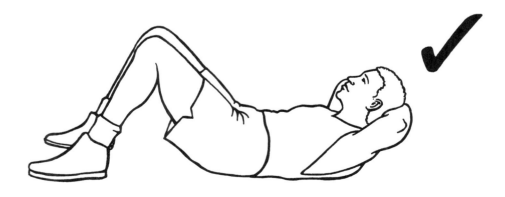

Slowly lift and lower your buttocks about 1 inch to perform reverse sit-ups. This is an effective alternative or addition to curl-ups. Avoid using momentum, lift buttocks straight to the ceiling. You can also do a crunch (combination curl-up and reverse sit-up). Simply curl-up as you simultaneously lift the buttocks. Slowly release and repeat.

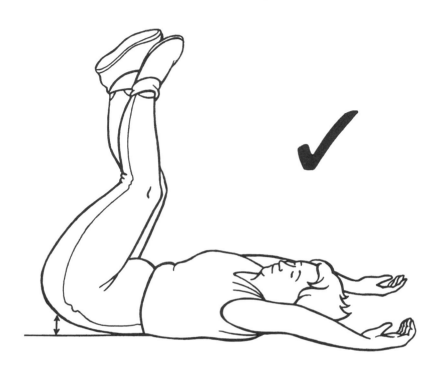

Slowly reaching to each side as you curl will work the oblique abdominal muscles. Return to neutral starting position after every contraction.

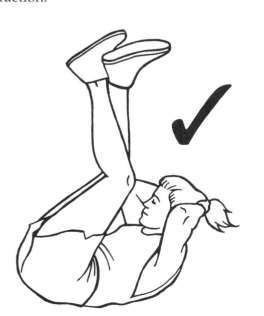

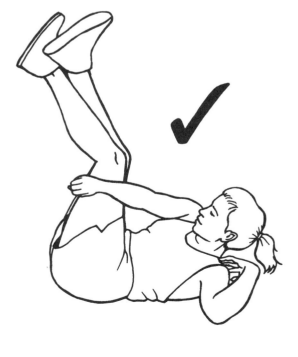

Hip and Thigh Calisthenics

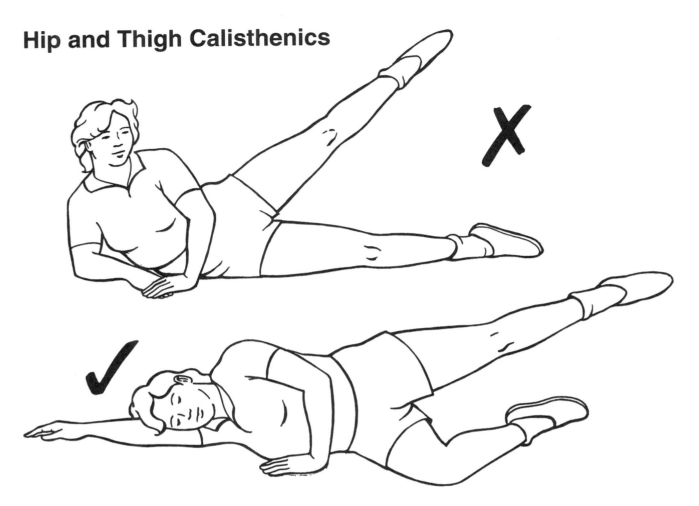

The side lying position can be used to work the abductors, adductors, and gluteals. You should not be up on your elbow because it limits range of motion and puts the spine in a misaligned position. The knee and toe should point forward so that the hip does not move out of line with the shoulder. Protect the lower back from arching by pulling the bottom knee forward. The top knee should remain slightly bent.

Lower Back Strengthening

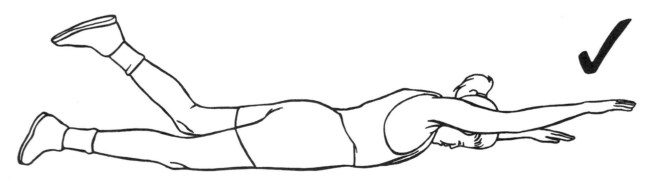

Keeping your head in line with your spine lift your right leg and left arm. Hold for 8 counts and then switch sides. As you advance lift both arms and both legs.

Hamstrings

To strengthen the hamstring, hold on to a sturdy object and pull the heel toward the buttocks. It is not necessary to come all the way up, just to about 90 degrees. Keep the support leg bent and the spine straight. Do enough repetitions to achieve overload. You will need a resistance band or an ankle weight to create overload on the muscle.

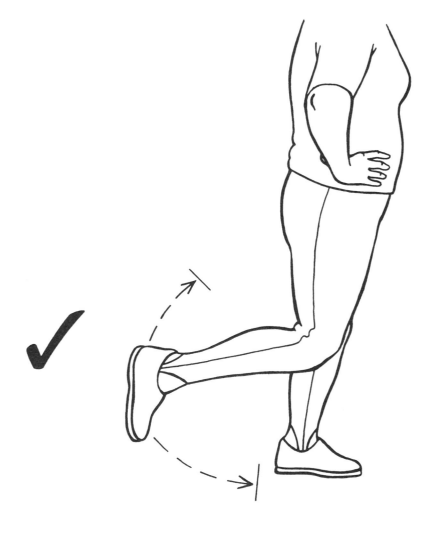

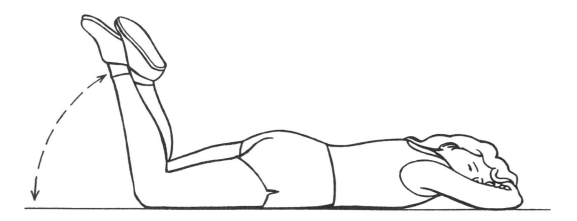

This exercise is excellent because it provides added resistance without equipment. Lie prone with the ankles crossed. Slowly pull the bottom foot toward the buttocks while resisting with the top foot. Do the reverse as you return to the starting position.

Muscles and Muscle Groups

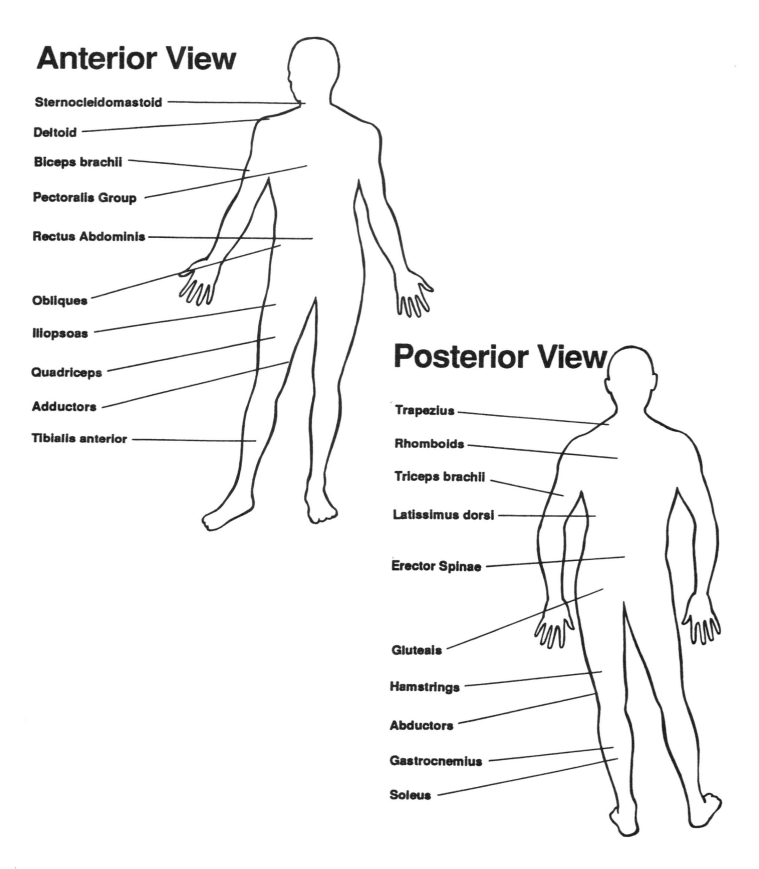

Anterior View

Sternocleidomastoid
Deltoid
Biceps brachii
Pectoralis Group
Rectus Abdominis
Obliques
Iliopsoas
Quadriceps
Adductors
Tibialis anterior

Posterior View

Trapezius
Rhomboids
Triceps brachii
Latissimus dorsi
Erector Spinae
Gluteals
Hamstrings
Abductors
Gastrocnemius
Soleus

Chapter Six

EXERCISE FOR SPECIAL POPULATIONS

Arthritis

The two basic forms of arthritis, osteoarthritis, and rheumatoid arthritis, have different causes but both result in pain within the joints. This pain leads to limited use and therefore decreased range of motion. Exercise programs need to carefully choose the appropriate amount and intensity of activity for each individual to reduce the severity of joint inflammation.

- A longer warm-up and cool-down is essential for arthritic patients in order to enhance joint lubrication and mobility
- Begin with low-intensity, frequent sessions.
- Decrease intensity and duration during bouts of pain.
- All joints should be moved through their range of motion at least once each day.
- Focus on proper posture and body alignment at all times.
- Use more isometric exercises. This means contracting the muscle without moving the joint.

Cardiovascular Disease

Persons with diagnosed cardiovascular disease can benefit greatly from rehabilitative exercise programs, stress reduction training, and nutrition education. Those patients who stay mobile after a cardiac event experience fewer complications and faster recoveries. These programs should only be conducted by qualified medical personnel with emergency equipment readily available. Often, after a patient has progressed successfully, their physician will give clearance for exercising outside the program. To maximize safety and to minimize a recurring cardiovascular event, patients should proceed very gradually, never exercise alone, and get specific recommendations from the physician and exercise physiologist with regard to frequency, intensity, and duration. Check to see whether any prescribed medications affect normal heart rate response to exercise. Patients should also be alert for symptoms such as shortness of breath, chest pain, nausea, dizziness or any other sign of discomfort.

Lower Back Pain

It is estimated that over 80% of us will experience back problems in our lifetimes. Our sedentary jobs and lifestyles are the primary cause. Must back injuries are the result of chronic degeneration over a long period of time. Low back pain is associated with excess body weight, smoking, and decreased physical activity. Poor posture, weak support (core) muscles, inadequate flexibility, improper body mechanics, pregnancy, and congenital problems can all contribute to back pain or injury.

There is no need to create a special exercise program for back pain because everyone should already be on a back program.. Even young people without back pain should follow a conservative, safe program such as the one in this book. Make sure you concentrate on strengthening the abdominals, hamstrings, and lower back and delete any contraindicated exercises from your workout. Prevent back pain before it starts. If you have mild low back pain following exercise apply ice. Some lower back problems can be very serious and thus require immediate medical care. If in doubt, consult your physician and a physical therapist.

- When standing for long periods, put one food on a stool to prevent swayback.
- When exercising always maintain the neutral pelvic position (see Chap. 5)
- Never exercise without warming up.
- Avoid head-forward positions in which the chin is tilted up.
- When lifting, use a wide stance and bend your knees and hips, not the waist. Keep the object close to your body. Avoid twisting. If the object is too heavy, get help!
- Do not slump when sitting, pull abdominals in, keep the spine straight and sit slightly forward.
- If your chair is too high, swayback is increased. When sitting, the knees should be even with the hips and the feet should be flat on the floor.
- Avoid leaning forward while sitting at a desk or table. If possible use a chair with arm rests to reduce the load on your spine.
- Wear comfortable, supportive shoes. Avoid high heels whenever possible.
- The best sleeping positions are on the side with knees bent or on the back with a support under the knees.
- Maintain ideal body weight.

Adhere to a regular exercise program paying particular attention to stretching and muscular balance and strength.

Diabetes Mellitus

The primary goal of exercise for diabetics is glucose regulation and reduced risk of heart disease. Physical exercise has been found to have an insulin-like effect on the body and thus facilitates the entry of glucose into the cells. Sometimes a patient gains better control of blood sugar levels or is able to decrease dosage of medication. Sporadic exercise is not effective, it must be regular. Exercise is appropriate only when performed under a physician's guidance and in combination with dietary and/or medical controls.

Simple carbohydrates, such as candy, fruit juice or sugar should be readily available at the exercise site in case hypoglycemia develops. Diabetics who use insulin should avoid injections into muscles which will be used directly in their workout. Working out at the same time each day may increase control. Good quality shoes and special attention to foot care are essential for diabetics. Specific exercise prescriptions will depend on each individual's health and fitness status as well as the advice of their doctor.

Hypertension

Regular aerobic exercise can lower both systolic and diastolic blood pressure by 10mmHg. Physical activity should be combined with weight loss, salt restriction and other dietary changes. Persons with high blood pressure should always obtain medical clearance before performing any type of exercise. A low to moderate intensity aerobic activity is best. Information about how the patient's medication will affect their heart rate should be provided by the physician. Hypertensive exercisers should avoid any static or isometric contractions which can raise blood pressure to dangerous levels. For example, straining to lift a heavy weight or pushing against a stationary object. Also, activities which require raised arm positions for long periods can increase pressure. Hypertensive patients should be coached to exhale on exertion and to avoid holding their breath. In addition, an extended warm-up, cool-down, and relaxation segment will increase the safety of the workout. Use of the RPE scale (Rating of Perceived Exertion) is the best way to monitor intensity (see Chap. 4). Many patients are able to decrease or discontinue medications after combining a regular exercise program with moderate weight loss and dietary changes.

Overweight or Obese Individuals

Although you can lose weight without exercising, a fitness program allows you to maintain lean mass and resting metabolic rate. A person should be judged obese by evaluation of both body fat percentage and body weight. Since movement and balance are limited to some degree, exercise is more difficult. Low-impact aerobic dance, walking, swimming, aqua-aerobics, or stationary cycling are all appropriate choices. Intensity should be set at 40% to 50% of maximal heart rate. Increase the intensity as fitness improves. Duration and frequency should slowly be increased to facilitate weight loss (ultimate goal: 30-50 minutes, 5-7 times/week or short bouts several times each day). A serious weight loss program will include aerobic exercise, strength training, dietary changes, and stress management. Developing a support system and addressing psychosocial issues are also very important. The maximal rate for safe weight loss is 1-2 lbs per week. Patience and diligence will eventually pay off where fad diets and magic potions will result in large swings of weight loss and weight gain. Lifestyle changes are the best way to lose weight and maintain the loss forever.

Pregnancy

With proper supervision, exercise for the pregnant woman can be extremely beneficial. The purpose is to maintain aerobic fitness and muscle strength, to prepare for labor and delivery, and to increase self-esteem and emotional health. Activities like swimming, aqua-aerobics, and stationary cycling are excellent. Walking is great if the temperature is not too high. Research shows that women who exercise regularly prior to pregnancy may be able to continue their normal program if they take precautions regarding temperature regulation and intensity and have no contraindications to exercise. The American College of Obstetricians and Gynecologists has determined guidelines and recommendations for exercising during pregnancy and during the postpartum period. These guidelines can be obtained from your obstetrician who can also give you individual advice.

Chapter Seven

NUTRITION FOR AN ACTIVE LIFESTYLE

The real news is not that a healthy diet is good for you. We all know that. The real news is that good nutrition may save your life! We now know that the right diet lowers a person's risk for many chronic diseases and enhances the benefits gained through regular exercise. Aerobic and strength workouts combined with proper nutrition will aid in weight control, help reduce calcium loss from bones, and reduce the negative effects of stress and anxiety. No matter what your personal goals for wellness are, a nutrition plan is essential. The good news is that you don't have to drastically change your lifestyle or go on one boring, impossible diet after another. A few carefully made changes can modify your nutritional habits for a lifetime of healthy eating.

Upsetting Food and Fat Facts

In one day in the United States we consume: 47 million hot dogs, 3 million gallons of ice cream, and 6 million pounds of chocolate.

In the past two decades, obesity rates have doubled, portion sizes have doubled, and the amount of food eaten outside of the home has doubled.

At the end of 2001 20.9% of Americans were obese and 7.9% were diabetic.

In 1910 the average adult consumed 70 pounds of refined sugar. Now that has risen to 150 pounds per year. Children and adolescents consume 275 pounds per year.

Of the children born in the year 2000, one in three will have diabetes.

Only one in five Americans eats the recommended five servings a day of fruits and vegetables. Twenty percent eat no fruit at all, and fifteen percent rarely eat a vegetable other than potatoes.

Only 13% of families with children get the minimum five servings of fruits and vegetables a day.

Ninety-seven percent of crash dieters not only regain the lost weight within one year but actually put on extra weight. This is particularly true when caloric intake falls to under 1,200 calories a day for men and 900 for women.

Girls who drink the most soda have five times the risk of broken bones.

Oxidative Stress and Phytonutrients

Living things require oxygen to survive. When we breathe oxygen we produce byproducts. This is similar to burning a fire in your fireplace. The word "burning" actually means reaction with oxygen. The byproduct is smoke which can cause damage if it becomes excessive. In your body the use of oxygen causes an abundance of free radicals. Free radicals are molecules which are missing an electron. They then roam around trying to steal an electron from healthy molecules causing damage wherever they go. This daily damage begins to break down your body bit by bit. The damaged cells become diseased and this can be the start of cancer or heart disease. This is called "oxidative stress". The free radicals can also damage your DNA which is your "blueprint" for producing more healthy cells. Research has now associated oxidative stress with almost every degenerative disease known, including cancer, heart disease, Alzheimers disease, macular degeneration, cataracts, wrinkling, and many others. Aging itself is the outcome of years of oxidative stress to all systems.

You must have antioxidants which come from fruits, vegetables, and grains to protect your body from the free radicals and repair the damage. These antioxidants are called phytonutrients or phytochemicals. They help protect the healthy cells from the free radicals by forming a hard coating or armor around the surface. There are thousands of phytonutrients which have been identified. Each color of fruits and vegetables has different nutrients. They all have important roles in human nutrition and in maintaining health. One apple has over 10,000 identified nutrients. These nutrients work in a delicate balance to perform all of the important functions in the cells of your body. You cannot get this from a manmade vitamin pill!

Whole Food Nutrition

The government and researchers have spent billions of dollars and tens of years trying to find a cure for heart disease, cancer, and other diseases. They have tried to discover what the one thing is in the orange that is good for you. After years of study we now know that it is the synergy of the whole orange that allows your body to function at its very best. Food should be eaten in the proportion that it was put on earth, not in fragmented, isolated vitamins or man-made elements. There is overwhelming evidence that people who eat a variety of raw fruits, raw vegetables, and unrefined grains have the least amount of disease. The problem is that very few humans actually consume the necessary amount and variety of these healthy foods.

After twenty years of never recommending any supplements I decided it is time to "think outside the box". The disease rates keep rising which is a serious call for action. What we are doing currently is not working. People know they should eat more fruits and vegetables but in reality it is not happening. That is why I recommend a few carefully chosen whole-food supplements, like omega-3 supplements and Juice Plus+® fruit and vegetable powders (see resource guide). My clients actually eat more fruits and vegetables and consume more fish once we get them on the right track and they see how much better they feel.

Benefits of a Diet High in Fruits and Vegetables

Helps control blood pressure

Enhances weight control

Decreased Incidence of Cancer (Lung, Oral, Larynx, Esophagus, Stomach, Pancreas, Cervix, Colorectal, Breast, Prostate)

Decreased Risk of Heart Disease and Stroke

Enhanced Immune System

Protect Eyesight (Macular Degeneration and Cataracts)

Combats Arthritis

Decreased Diseases of the Digestive System

Decreases Homocysteine which is a risk factor for coronary artery disease, heart attack and stroke and is associated with many other diseases.

Should I Take Man-Made Vitamin and Mineral Supplements?

Researchers are beginning to understand that vitamin supplements cannot make up for a poor diet and that supplements have not been shown to cure any disease. With so much fortification it seems easier to overdose and actually increase the risk of disease.

Certain segments of the populations with specific needs may need supplements if they cannot consume or absorb enough whole food sources. Examples include: Pregnant women who do not consume enough folic acid, elderly people who cannot absorb enough B12, and people who stay indoors a lot and cannot make their own Vitamin D. You should never go against what your physician recommends.

Having said the above, the most common supplements consumed include vitamin E and C. Vitamin E supplements can increase the risk of heart attacks and strokes, and studies of vitamin C supplements consistently fail to show any benefits. Vitamin A supplements increase the risk of osteoporosis and have been shown to double the risk of bone fractures. Iron is an oxidant which in quantities too high can increase the risk of heart disease. Iron deficiency is currently very rare. Dr. Caballero (Director of the Center for Human Nutrition at Johns Hopkins University) reports that "large, rigorous studies that were supposed to show that individual vitamins prevented disease ended up showing the opposite. Those who took the vitamins actually had more of the disease it was meant to prevent." Two studies on Beta-carotene and Vitamin E were stopped early because the groups getting the vitamins had a higher death rate than the groups getting the placebo.

The secret seems to be in the synergy of how vitamins and minerals found naturally in the foods we eat work together. Dr. Caballero concludes "If you eat junk food every day, vitamins are the least of your problems," he said. "You cannot replace a healthy diet. We don't know what ingredient in a healthy diet is responsible for which condition. We do know that people who consume five servings or more of fruits and vegetables have less disease. But we don't know which ingredient. We tried beta carotene, vitamin E and antioxidants, and they didn't work."

Changes in the Food Supply

The tomato that our grandparents consumed may not have the same nutritional content as the one that is picked before it is fully ripe across the country and then shipped by truck to be sold one week later. The chemicals that are part of our soil, pesticides, herbicides, antibiotics, hormones, radiation: these are all elements that our ancestors did not have to encounter in their food. Even though we may eat exactly the same diet as someone did 50 years ago, the nutrient and toxin content in the food may be very different.

VIP—VERY IMPORTANT POINT

You cannot prevent disease or slow the progression of any disease without an adequate intake and variety of raw fruits, vegetables, and grains. This must come from whole food sources. If you do not get enough in your diet, add a whole food supplement like *Juice Plus+*® (see resource guide). This product has been classified as a food, not a vitamin or a drug. It is simply juiced fruits and vegetables in a powder form. It is a convenient way to get extra fruits and vegetables into your diet. How is Juice Plus+® made? The 17 fruits and vegetables are juiced. The sugar, sodium, some fiber, and water are removed at a low temperature to produce fruit and vegetable powders. This process allows the thousands of phytonutrients and antioxidants to remain intact. It comes in capsules, chewables, and gummies. It is certified as pesticide free. This is one of the few supplements that I recommend because it has a large body of primary, peer-reviewed research to show that it works like the actual whole fruits and vegetables. My own family has used Juice Plus+® for six years with outstanding results.

Scientific, original, peer-reviewed research on Juice Plus+®

- significantly raises the levels of key antioxidants

- lowers the levels of lipid peroxides (a measure of oxidative stress)

- significantly improves major immune functions (T-cell, B-cell and natural killer cell activity and cytokine levels)

- significantly reduces DNA damage

- significantly improves blood circulation following a high-fat meal

- significantly reduces serum homocysteine levels as it raises the level of antioxidants in the bloodstream.

What Should I Eat?

The information in this book is intended as a general guideline for healthy people. If you have any medical conditions or are taking any medications it is important to consult a registered dietician and your physician for specific advice. Remember that there are no "bad" foods, only foods that should be strictly limited or used in moderation. If your favorite food is high in fat and sugar you will need to save it for very special occasions or possibly decrease the quantity. If you really savor the taste you may not need such a large portion. Go for quality – not quantity!

Carbohydrates

Carbohydrates are the most important nutrient for exercising muscles and are needed for optimal brain and central nervous system function. The recommended amount of carbohydrate is 55-60% of your total caloric intake (4 to 6 grams per kg of body weight). People who exercise for longer than one hour every day should consume 65% carbohydrates or more. Carbohydrates are necessary nutrients but it is important to consume the right kind. Refined sugars and starches have little nutritional value and are quickly absorbed and stored as fat. Because these sugary foods are digested so quickly they overload the blood with glucose. Over time consumption of high amounts of simple carbohydrates and starch leads to diabetes and other diseases.

Complex carbohydrates are foods that are left in their whole state. Whole grains, potatoes, corn, rice, fruits and vegetables. They still have the vitamins, minerals and fiber and take much longer to be broken down. The sugars are released much more slowly into the bloodstream avoiding excess glucose in the blood.

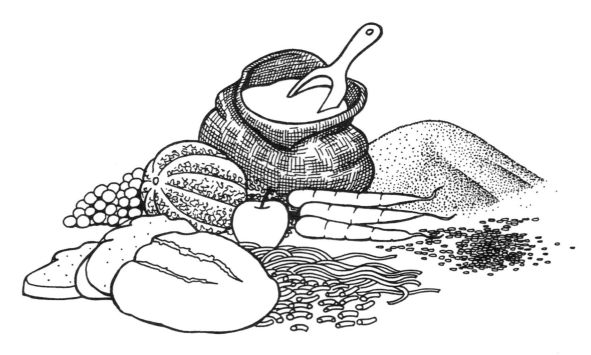

Foods High in Complex Carbohydrates

Protein

The job of protein is to build and repair body tissues, including muscles, tendons, and ligaments. It is also necessary for the synthesis of hormones, enzymes, and antibodies, as well as fluid transport and energy. It is very rare in developed nations, especially the United States for there to be deficiencies in protein intake. Most of us eat too much and choose poor quality sources. Research suggests an active adult needs 0.8 to 1.0 grams of protein per kg of body weight. Others suggest that we need even less. Excess protein puts stress on the digestive tract, kidneys, and liver. Too much protein from meat sources causes an excess of Uric acid. In order to neutralize this acid the body steals calcium from bones and stores in the body, leaching the body of calcium. Some nutritionists believe the reason we need such a high intake of calcium is because of our higher than needed intake of protein. Some even implicate the rise in osteoporosis with the increase in protein in our diets. The Nutrition Committee of the Council on Nutrition, Physical activity, and Metabolism of the American Heart Association state, "High-protein diets are not recommended because they restrict healthful foods that provide essential nutrients and do not provide the variety of foods needed to adequately meet nutritional needs. Individuals who follow these diets are therefore at risk for compromised vitamin and mineral intake, as well as potential cardiac, renal, bone, and liver abnormalities overall."

You can easily get the protein you need from fruits, vegetables, soy foods, beans, grains, seeds, and nuts. Fish is an excellent source as well. Avoid protein supplements and high-protein energy bars. If you choose to eat beef and poultry choose low-fat varieties and do not consume the skin. Free range and grass-fed are best. Free range eggs are also a good choice as they have a higher ratio of omega-3 fatty acids. Dairy products should be skim and organic.

Fat

Fat is the primary fuel you use for light to moderate-intensity exercise. You should not consume more than 35% of your calories from fat. The essential fatty acids provided by the fat in your diet are important for maintaining healthy cell membranes, healthy skin, making hormones, and transporting certain vitamins. The type of fat is the important thing.

Reduce Saturated Fat and Cholesterol

Animal food is the primary source for saturated fat in the diet. Fat on beef, pork, veal, the skin on poultry, dairy products like cheese, lard, and butter, are all common sources of saturated fats. It is also found in palm oil, palm kernel oil, and coconut oil. There is overwhelming research showing that diets high in saturated fats raise the risk of heart disease, stroke, and many forms of cancer.

Avoid Trans-Fat or Hydrogenated Fat

These are fats which have been altered to make them have a longer shelf life. They are very damaging and are mostly found in cookies, cakes, crackers, and other highly processed foods. Trans fatty acids are very hard for your body to break down. They stick together causing fatty deposits in the arteries and the liver. Like saturated fat they are associated with a higher incidence of heart disease and stroke.

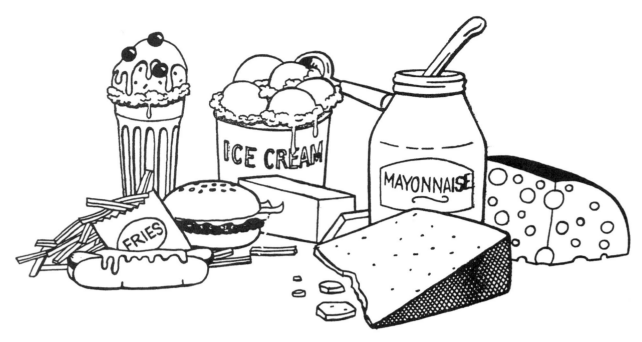

Foods with a High Fat Content

Cooking Oil

The best choices are monounsaturated fats like olive oil and canola oil. The best olive oil is virgin or extra virgin because it is the least oxidized. Extra oleic safflower or extra oleic sunflower oil are also good. Avoid regular sunflower oil, safflower oil and corn oil because they are too high in omega-6 fatty acids. Real butter is better than margarines (trans-fat). Remember that all oils are equally high in calories.

Omega-3 Fatty Acids

Every cell in our body needs omega-3 fatty acids to function optimally. We cannot manufacture them ourselves so they must be ingested. The omega-6 fatty acids are also essential but our modern diets contain plenty of this oil. During the last century people in developed countries like the United States have eliminated almost all omega-3 fatty acids from their diet. Where we used to have a ratio of one omega-6 to one omega-3 we now have a ratio of 15 omega-6 to one omega-3.

What do omega-3 fatty acids do in the body? They help control energy production in the cell and they are the building blocks of your cell membranes, controlling what comes in and out of the cell.

Research has discovered that this depletion of omega-3's has had a very negative effect on our bodies, in particular the brain and the heart. The rise in heart disease and depression has directly paralleled this decrease in omega-3 consumption. Other diseases related to this deficiency are rheumatoid arthritis, diabetes, postpartum depression, cancer, obesity, asthma, attention disorders, and aggression/hostility in teenagers.

There used to be an abundance of omega-3 fatty acids in the food supply especially in populations that ate fish and wild game. When cows and chickens were allowed to roam free and eat grass, the meat and eggs had a much higher content of omega-3's. Because our food supply has changed drastically people consume little or no omega-3's. Salmon that is farm-raised has no chance to eat the algae which makes wild, fatty fish high in this essential nutrient. Fish have also been contaminated with environmental pollutants like mercury and PCB's which makes it less desirable to eat the amounts needed to get adequate omega-3s.

VIP-VERY IMPORTANT POINT

Increase omega-3 fatty acids in your diet and decrease omega-6 containing oils (corn oil, safflower oil and sunflower oil).

Good Sources of omega-3s are:

Oily fish (salmon, mackerel, tuna)

Fortified eggs or eggs from free-range/grass fed chickens

Wild Game

Soy Foods/Tofu

Walnuts

Flax and Hemp Seeds

Flaxseed Oil

High Quality/Purified Fish Oil Supplements (See resource guide for more information and check with your physician before consuming a supplement)

Other Important Nutritional Concerns

Is It That Simple?
The Truth about Metabolism, Appetite, and Weight Loss

Our lifestyles include sedentary jobs, video games, hours of television, loss of physical education programs and recess in schools, and a lack of playgrounds and safe neighborhoods to play in. On average, Americans lose about five to seven pounds of lean tissue every decade while gaining about 10 additional pounds of fat per decade. Less muscle leads to a lower metabolic rate. In fact our muscle loss is largely responsible for the 2-5% per decade reduction in metabolism.

Studies are showing that weight loss is much more complicated than we once believed. Some people respond much faster than others to dietary and activity changes. Genetic factors are extremely important in determining our body type and response to weight loss interventions. To avoid frustration we must be aware of this component and learn to recognize that what works for each individual may vary.

Although the research is in its infancy the following components have been found to influence appetite and weight control: genetic factors, calcium levels, insulin, leptin, high intake of fructose, stress hormones, serotonin depletion, surging levels of Neuropeptide Y, and differing numbers of taste buds. Being overweight is not a character flaw or weakness. Seek out a physician and registered dietician who have studied these issues. Understanding these complex physiological processes can relieve guilt and help steer you toward effective weight management solutions.

Resting metabolism is extremely important in the weight control equation. Researchers believe that it may be possible to raise metabolism, especially by increasing muscle mass with strength training and possibly with long term aerobic exercise. Excess calories (carbohydrates, protein, or fat) will be stored as fat so the important thing is to find exercise activities that you will do. All physical exercise helps to burn excess calories. You may burn more total calories with high-intensity activity but low-intensity is better for unfit or overweight individuals and may produce fewer injuries. There is nothing wrong with very fit people taking advantage of high-intensity aerobic activities to burn more calories in a shorter amount of time.

For optimal weight loss professionals recommend combining a decrease in caloric intake with an increase in physical activity. In other words, eat less and exercise more to achieve gradual permanent weight loss. This is called "The Balance Equation". Too few calories can also be a problem. Your body must have the fuel it needs to function and perform.

The Balance Equation for Weight Control

ENERGY INTAKE = ENERGY OUTPUT

(food or calories)   **(resting metabolism and**
                                              physical activity)

Hydration and Fluid Intake

Everyone should drink 6 to 8 glasses (8 ounces) of water each day. Adequate fluid intake is necessary to replace fluids lost through metabolism, daily activity and vigorous exercise. The amount lost depends on many factors including environmental temperature, humidity, and your ability to dissipate heat. Drink water before, during and after your workout. If you exercise longer than one hour a sports drink is recommended (5 to 8% carbohydrate with 100 mg of sodium).

Guidelines for Exercise Fluid Replacement

Consume 8 to 16 ounces of fluid at least one hour before the start of exercise.

Consume 4 to 8 ounces of fluid every 10-15 minutes during the workout.

Consume 16-24 ounces during the 30 minutes after exercise even if you do not feel thirsty.

Fiber

Fiber refers to the components of plant cell walls that are not digested by human intestinal enzymes. It is also called "roughage" or "bulk". When whole grains are processed or refined much of the fiber is removed and many of the nutrients are lost. Fiber adds bulk to the diet, absorbs water in the intestine and produces larger, softer stools that are easily eliminated. This decreases the time that cancer causing agents are in contact with the lining of the large intestine and colon. This also inhibits the absorption of toxins into the bloodstream. People who consume a high-fiber diet have less colon cancer, heart disease, cholesterol problems, and gallstones. Soluable fiber forms a gel as it moves through the digestive system interfering with the absorption of cholesterol. Oat bran, oatmeal, barley, rice bran, apples, oranges, strawberries, prunes, carrots, corn broccoli, lentils, navy beans and pinto beans all contain soluable fiber. Fiber of any kind is also great for weight loss as it fills the stomach and decreases appetite.

Conditions associated with low-fiber diets are chronic constipation, diverticulitis, irritable colon syndrome, Crohn's Disease, colitis, and blood clots in veins and lungs. Cancer, heart disease, diabetes, and kidney problems have all been linked to low-fiber diets.

VIP- VERY IMPORTANT POINT

The optimum diet should have about 25-40 grams of fiber a day. Fruits, vegetables, legumes (beans), nuts, whole grain breads, cereals and rice are great choices.

Sodium

Americans consume two to four teaspoons of salt a day – this adds up to 15 pounds of salt each year! The American Heart Association recommends ½ to 1 teaspoon each day.

Alcohol

First the negative side: Alcoholic beverages are low in nutrient content and high in calories. According to the American Institute for Cancer Research, there is convincing evidence that alcoholic drinks increase the risk of cancers of the mouth, pharynx, larynx, and esophagus. The risk of upper respiratory tract cancers is greatly increased if drinkers also smoke. Alcohol also increases the risk of liver cancer and probably increases the risk for colon, rectal, and breast cancers. Although it may be true that alcohol can lower risk for coronary heart disease, it increases risk in so many other areas (high blood pressure, stroke, birth defects, inflammation of the pancreas, damage to the brain and heart, malnutrion osteoporosis, accidents, violence, and suicide) it might not be worth taking a chance

Now the positive: Moderate alcohol consumption is associated with a decreased risk of heart disease and stroke. Alcohol causes LDL to decrease and HDL to increase. It also aids in dissolving clots that have already formed. Many alcohol beverages, including red wine and beer have powerful antioxidants that reduce oxidative stress. Moderate drinkers also have lower levels of C-reactive protein which is a marker of inflammation in the body. Moderate drinkers also had less risk of dying of heart disease than non-drinkers or heavy drinkers.

Be a Smart Consumer

Try to buy foods that contain ingredients you recognize or would use at home.

Stay on the perimeter of the grocery store. This is where the fresh, whole food is sold.

Avoid products containing the following ingredients: partially hydrogenated oils, artificial sweeteners (aspartame), nitrites, nitrates, artificial colors, sulfites, potassium bromate, and brominated vegetable oil.

Any diet book or plan that promises large decreases in weight in a short amount of time should be avoided.

The following terms all mean one thing – sugar! Brown sugar, honey, dextrose, maltose, lactose, fructose, rock sugar, and corn syrup. No one sugar is healthier or better than another, they are all simply empty calories. Most of us eat way too much.

Check serving sizes. Most of us eat much more than a typical serving. A small bag of chips might actually be 2 ½ or more servings. It is a sneaky trick! You must multiply the servings by 2.5 to get your total intake.

Protein, fat, and carbohydrate are sometimes listed by weight, not percentage of total calories. This can be very deceiving since fat has more than twice the calories per gram than protein or carbohydrate. In the example below, milk that is 2% fat by weight is actually 38% fat by calories. You don't need to carry your calculator to the store when you shop. Just be aware of the type and amount of fat in the foods you normally purchase. Make substitutions for the high-fat (saturated and trans fat) foods.

Reading Labels

1 gram of fat	=9 kilocalories
1 gram of protein	=4 kilocalories
1 gram of carbohydrate	=4 kilocalories
1 gram of alcohol	=7 kilocalories

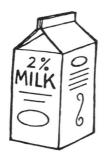

Example: 2% Milk (information from the nutritional label)

1 serving (1 cup) = 120 total calories

5 grams of fat X 9 calories = 45 calories from fat

45 (calories of fat) divided by 120 (total calories)= 38% of calories from fat

Ideas for Snacks

Raw Fruits (Dip in Yogurt or Peanut Butter)

Raw Vegetables (Dip in Hummus, Salsa, Bean Dip or Peanut Butter)

Yogurt (We make parfaits with layers of fruit and high fiber cereal)

Cheese Slices on Whole Wheat Crackers

Peanut Butter on Whole Wheat Crackers

Nuts

Air Popped Popcorn

Hard Boiled Eggs (boil on the weekend and keep them in the fridge)

Whole Grain Cereals

Dried Fruit

Smoothie (yogurt, soy beverage, or skim organic milk with ripe bananas and frozen fruit)

Osteoporosis

Bones are living tissues, constantly being remodeled and reacting to hormonal changes, nutrition, and stressors applied to them. Osteoporosis is a disease in which low bone mass and deterioration of bone structure causes bones to be weak, porous, brittle, and susceptible to fracture. At highest risk are Asian and Caucasian females who are relatively thin and sedentary, postmenopausal women without estrogen support, and those with a family history of osteoporosis. Black females are at lower risk probably because of greater bone mass. Men can develop osteoporosis but it usually shows up much later in life.

VIP - VERY IMPORTANT POINT

Researchers are beginning to realize that the main cause of osteoporosis is a high intake of acidic food, mainly protein. The higher the intake of protein, the more uric acid is produced which must be neutralized by calcium from bones and teeth. Animal products and processed foods also contain high levels of phosphorous which also has to be neutralized with calcium. Osteoporosis is linked with kidney disorders because of the high stress on the kidneys to eliminate the protein. The answer is to eat a diet high in fruits and vegetables which have a high calcium to phosphorous ratio. The calcium is much more available and easy to absorb and prevents leaching of calcium from bones and teeth. Try to increase tofu, soy products (processed with calcium sulphate or calcium chloride), bok choy, broccoli, kale, turnip greens, parsley, mustard greens, and endive.

Avoid These to Prevent Osteoporosis

Tobacco – Lowers hormone levels, thereby accelerating bone loss. Stopping smoking at any age slows bone loss.

High Caffeine Intake – Increases the amount of calcium excreted in the urine, depriving the bones of calcium they need. Carbonated sodas have phosphates which cause loss of calcium from bones and teeth.

Alcohol Consumption – Suppresses bone tissue formation.

Excessive Dieting – Hurts the bones by depriving the body of important nutrients, including calcium. Eating disorders can also affect bone health.

Excessive Physical Activity – Can cause bone loss by depressing hormone levels, evident when a female exerciser begins to miss her normal menstrual periods (amenorrhea).

Ways to Prevent Osteoporosis

Consume a calcium-rich diet – Calcium is essential to healthy bones. This is extremely important during the teen years and early adulthood when we build our peak bone density, but also throughout our lives. Vegetable sources are best. Include: skim milk, yogurt, cheese, calcium-fortified juice, tofu, soy products (processed with calcium sulphate or calcium chloride), bok choy, broccoli, kale, turnip greens, canned sardines, salmon with bones, calcium supplements as needed.

Vitamin D – Necessary for our bodies to absorb calcium. Sources: sunshine, dairy products, supplements.

Consult a physician – Learn about your risk for osteoporosis and the recommended treatment.

Eating Disorders

With the emphasis in this country on beauty and possessing a perfect physique it is very difficult to maintain a healthy attitude concerning body image, eating, and weight control. Eating disorders are an outward sign of emotional disturbances. Various eating disorders have become more prominent in recent years, especially among teenagers and young adults. Typically, but not exclusively, eating disorders are diagnosed in females of at least average intelligence but better than average achievement from middle to upper socioeconomic classes. The pressure to achieve and to control escalates into a compulsion to be perfect in everything: grades, possessions, looks, relationships, etc. Eating disorders can take several forms including Anorexia Nervosa, Bulimia, Binge Disorders and combinations of these. The top priority is to attain professional medical help for victims of eating disorders.

Eat to live and not live to eat.

Benjamin Franklin, 1733

Chapter Eight

Injury Prevention and Treatment

Carefully planning and executing your fitness plan should make injuries non-existent. For the sake of completeness and recognizing that accidents do occur, the following information has been included.

The RICE Treatment for Fitness Injuries

Several things happen when ice is applied to injured tissue. The blood vessels constrict decreasing blood flow to the area. This reduces bleeding and therefore swelling. Cold also acts as an anesthetic, controlling pain and relieving muscle spasms. Ice slows down metabolism around the injury slowing the release of histamine that increases inflammation and swelling. You can use ice packs, ice baths, or ice massages. Apply as quickly as possible.

REST	Stop immediately when you feel pain
ICE	Apply ice for 20-30 minutes several times per day
COMPRESSION	Firmly wrap the injured area (not too tight) with elastic or compression bandages. Bandages should reach from the largest area below the injury to the largest area above the injury.
ELEVATION	Raise the affected area level with or slightly above the heart to encourage blood flow to and from the injury.

Heat should never be applied too soon or it will increase swelling and bleeding into tissues. At least 72 hours after the injury use heat (warm, not hot) to increase blood flow to the area. Oxygen delivery is increased and waste products are removed. Apply 2-3 times a day for 20-30 minutes at a time. After 2 or 3 days you can alternate cold with heat (contrast bath). Hot for 1-2 minutes (96 to 98 degrees) and then cold (55 to 64 degrees) for 1-2 minutes. Repeat several times and finish with cold for 5 minutes. In all cases, if pain becomes worse or persists for a prolonged period, seek medical attention immediately. Progress slowly upon resuming your activity.

Common Injuries Associated with Exercise

Muscle Soreness (Delayed Onset Muscle Soreness)

Breakdown and repair of muscle results in stronger muscle, therefore, mild muscle soreness may be a good sign. Muscle soreness usually occurs when you begin an exercise regimen, perform eccentric contractions (lengthening the muscle), or you change your normal fitness routine. Microscopic tears in the muscle or connective tissue may require several days of rest for tissue repair and rebuilding. Severe soreness is unnecessary. The key is prevention. Progress slowly. Start with low repetition and low intensity and make sure you warm-up and cool-down properly. Avoid ballistic movements and stretches. If you do become sore it will usually last 24 to 48 hours regardless of what you do to treat it. Sometimes repeating mild exercise the following day and then performing slow, static stretches will relieve some of the discomfort. Massage and warm baths may also help.

Shin Splints

Inflammation or pain occurring where the muscles and tendons attach to bones can cause pain in the front portion of the lower leg. This can result from poorly fitted shoes, and improper running surface or a program which is too intense. An imbalance between the gastrocnemius and the tibialis anterior may also contribute to shin problems. Other causes of shin splints include: a lowered arch (flat feet), decreased flexibility in the Achilles tendon, irritated membranes, tearing of muscle where it attaches to bone, hairline or stress fracture of the bone, or other factors. The best treatment is RICE, however, stopping the aggravating activity and switching to a low impact activity for a while may allow time for healing while maintaining fitness. See a medical doctor to rule out fractures.

Knee Problems

Pain in the knee can be very difficult to diagnose. Many times it is the result of overuse, poorly fitted shoes, improper running surfaces, or biomechanical problems. Using proper progression, avoiding uneven surfaces, making sure your muscles are balanced, and not allowing injuries to become chronic will help prevent serious knee problems. Always see a physician and physical therapist if pain persists.

Ankle Problems

Ankle sprains are the most common ankle injury. Prevention includes strengthening exercises, adequate warm-up, proper footwear and ankle bracing. Activities that require quick changes of direction or exercises performed on an uneven surface may increase the chance of sprains. If an ankle injury should occur the ankle should be iced immediately and medical treatment should be sought.

Achilles' Tendon

Achilles' tendonitis, which is inflammation of the sheath around the Achilles' tendon, can cause severe pain and is a frequent complaint of distance runners. Usually, improper shoes or lack of flexibility are the culprit and stretching or ice and rest are the treatment.

Side Stitch

This is a sharp pain in the side beneath the ribs. Possible causes for this pain include: an oxygen deficiency, gas pains, spasms of the diaphragm or an improper warm-up. Often it will disappear if you lower the intensity of your activity, take slow, deep breaths, or bend toward the stitch and press gently on the painful area.

Heat Injuries

In extremely hot temperatures or high humidity you need to be very careful to avoid heat cramps, heat exhaustion, and heat stroke. Heat cramps are the mildest heat-stress problem. Symptoms include muscle twitches and cramping in the arms, legs, and abdomen. If you experience any of the following symptoms you may be suffering from heat exhaustion and should cool off and drink fluids containing potassium: headache, severe fatigue, nausea, low urinary output, clamminess, weak and rapid pulse, dizziness. Hot, dry, flushed skin, incoherent behavior, inability to perspire or seizures can be related to heat stroke and thus medical attention is required immediately. If not treated, heat stroke can be fatal. To insure hydration drink 8-10 eight ounce glasses of water per day.

Cardiovascular Problems

Half of all cardiac deaths occur in the first hour of the onset of symptoms. You should seek medical attention immediately if you experience any of the following symptoms.

- Pain or pressure in the chest, arm, or throat

- Abnormal heart activity like fluttering, jumping, or palpitations in the chest or throat.

- Nausea, dizziness, sudden lack of coordination, confusion, cold sweating, fainting, or any other unusual symptom that you cannot explain.

Prevention Is the Key

Progress slowly until you reach a maintenance level. Exercising too frequently or for long durations may predispose you to injuries. Never "work through the pain". If you feel any discomfort do not continue. Seek the appropriate treatment and do not resume the activity until the problem is corrected.

Chapter Nine

EXERCISE AND STRESS THE MIND-BODY CONNECTION

Stress! We all have it. It can be positive or negative. However, too much of any stress can seriously affect physical and mental well being. I find that my clients have trouble sticking with exercise and dietary changes until they have dealt with their chronic stress. We now know much more about the "mind-body connection". It has been estimated that 60-70% of all diseases are in some way stress-related. 89% of adults report that they experience high stress levels and 75 to 90% of doctor visits are stress-related. To achieve total wellness we must address all aspects of our lives and strive for balance.

What does Stress do to Your Body?

The Fight or Flight Syndrome

Immediate Effects

> Increased breathing rate
> Increased heart rate and blood pressure
> Fats and sugars are released into your blood stream
> Increased blood clotting
> Increased cortisol

Long-term Effects

> Increased cholesterol
> Increased blood pressure
> Increased homocysteine (a measure of inflammation)
> Leads to constricted arteries and abnormal heart rhythms

Compromised Immune System
Poor memory
Increased drug abuse and alcoholism
Increased obesity and overweight
Stomach and digestive problems
Grinding teeth, nervous habits

Stress Vulnerability

Recent research has focused on "stress vulnerability". Two people may have the same stressors and problems but one gets sick and one stays well. Why is this? Changing our physical and mental response to the stress is what is important. Research shows that people who adhere to the following behaviors stay well and develop fewer stress-related diseases.

- Eat a balanced and nutritious diet.

- Exercise regularly

- Get plenty of rest and sleep.

- Avoid abuse of alcohol, tobacco, or drugs.

- Organize your life and have a plan for your finances.

- Surround yourself with positive people and friends you can count on in times of stress.

- Take control of situations and make firm commitments to projects you care about.

- Nurture your spiritual life.

- Laugh often: See the humor in every situation.

- Learn to get rid of anger, hostility, and resentment. Get professional help if necessary.

- Focus on concerns that have a solution instead of worrying about things you cannot change.

- Be assertive and make your needs known to others in an honest and polite manner.

- Exercise your brain: Read, do puzzles, play games, visit museums......

- Travel and see the world....Go on vacation!

- Be adventurous....Keep the creative spark

- Get a pet…..Walk your dog whether you have one or not!

- Design your castle: Your home should reflect the true you and give you serenity.

- Keep romance in your life.!

- Volunteer …Takes the focus off of yourself and helps others.

Exercise and Stress Management

Exercise is one of the best ways to control and reduce the stress in your life. Activity provides a diversion, getting you away from the source of stress to clear your mind and to sort through the problems. Regular exercise makes you look better and feel better about yourself. Others will notice your improved self-concept. Physiological changes that occur with long-term, regular activity provide more strength, endurance, and energy to cope with difficult situations. Muscular tension which builds up throughout a stressful day is easily released with aerobic activity and stretching.

These physiological changes are also consistent with disease prevention. Exercise can reverse or improve many of the health problems that are related to stress. Benefits can include decreased high blood pressure, lowered cholesterol, reduced stress hormones, improved sleeping patterns, improvement in depression and mood, lower body fat, and lower body weight.

Stress Reduction and Relaxation

Mindful Breathing – A simple deep breath or two can promote an immediate relaxation response. Deep breathing should not happen in your chest but in the abdominal area. Your diaphragm will lower and your abdominals will push out. Take time out for sixty seconds when things get tense. Take time to close your eyes and focus on your breathing. When your To Do List sneaks into your mind, just go back and focus on your breathing.

Meditation – Follow the instructions for mindful breathing but choose an object or word to focus on. Empty your mind of everything else. And just slowly repeat the word mentally, over and over again.

Mental Imagery – During or after the final stretch of your workout clear your mind and focus on one single image. This could be a shape, a color, your favorite place or anything you associate with quiet and peace. It is simply a "mental vacation." It takes practice to avoid letting your mind wander to other things. Combine this technique with slow, deep breathing.

Visualization – By using mental pictures you can change attitudes and behaviors. Improve your organization by imagining what your office will look like when it is in order or improve your posture by imagining puppet strings attached to the top of your head and shoulders. Athletes are very successful in improving their performance using visualization training.

Progressive Muscle Relaxation – Progressive relaxation trains your muscles to release tension as it builds up instead of storing it throughout the day. Lie in a comfortable position (on your back or on your side with bent knees). Close your eyes. Start by taking several deep, slow breaths. Now, as you breath in you are going to tense a muscle or muscle group, as you exhale let the muscle relax. Focus on how different it feels in the tense state versus the relaxed state.

Follow this sequence:

Inhale, flex your right foot.

Exhale, let it relax.

Inhale, flex your left foot.

Exhale, let it go.

Repeat with the following contractions, inhaling and exhaling slowly each time.

Flex your feet and tense calf muscles.

Tighten both legs and press them together.

Tighten the thighs.

Tighten the buttocks.

Pull in the abdominal area and flatten the back.

Tense your chest and shrug the shoulders.

Clench your fists and press your arms into the floor.

Close your eyes tight and contract your jaw and facial muscles.

If you still feel tension in an area continue contacting and relaxing until the tightness disappears.

Massage – Treat yourself to massage therapy. Research demonstrates many valuable health and stress-reducing benefits.

Be Good to Yourself

This is it! You only get one body and one life. Treat them right. You may need to make an appointment with yourself to find time for exercise or for something that gives you pleasure. Other tactics include seeking help with time management, delegating responsibility and learning to say no. Seek opportunities that offer personal growth and discovery. Remember that you are special. Focus on relaxation, enjoyment, and health.

Summary

The Total Workout

You now have the necessary information to design a safe and effective exercise program. Below is a summary of the components of a total workout (approximately 1 hour). If your time is limited, you can always warm-up, perform 20 minutes of aerobic activity, cool down and stretch. Muscle work can be done on alternate days (Or see 'Exercise Lite' in Chapter 4). This fitness routine will fit easily into your lunch or other free time. On extremely busy days remember that something is better than nothing, a 15 minute walk or 10 minutes of strengthening exercises while you watch the news will be beneficial and help to maintain your fitness level.

Circulatory/Thermal Warm-up (4 to 10 minutes)

Purpose: To increase core temperature and blood flow to the working muscles, increase metabolic function, speed nerve transmission, and prevent injuries. Perform general activities at a low intensity level until you are perspiring lightly. On cold days this will take longer.

Optional Stretching Warm-up (1 to 3 minutes)

Purpose: Mild static stretching to prepare for the activity. Never stretch cold!

Aerobic Activity (20 to 60 minutes)

Purpose: To maintain rhythmic, continuous exercise for at least 20 minutes. Participate in aerobic activity at least 3 times per week, more for weight loss. Include interval training once a week.

Cool Down (3 to 10 minutes)

Purpose: Perform low-intensity, general movements until the heart rate falls below 120 beats per minute (100 beats if you are over 50 years old). Keep the feet and legs moving so that the blood will be pumped back toward the heart.

Muscular Strength and Endurance (10 to 30 minutes)

Purpose: Sufficient work on each muscle or muscle group to create overload. The goals are strength, endurance, and muscular balance. Concentrate on strengthening the weaker muscles. This segment can come before or after the aerobic activity but must follow a circulatory/thermal warm-up. Calisthenics, stretchy bands, or weights can all be effective with proper form.

Stretching and Relaxation (5 to 15 minutes)

Purpose: You must be warm. Perform static stretching for each joint designed to maintain or increase flexibility. Hold 10 to 30 seconds. Include relaxation and breathing exercises to release stress, anxiety, and muscular tension.

RECIPE FOR MAXIMAL HEALTH

Goals for a Happy and Healthy Life

To remain functional and independent until the day I die.....
To practice preventive health-care/ not "only when I'm sick or hurting healthcare".....
To make exercise, rest, and proper nutrition a normal part of my day.....
To recognize that stress is normal; however, I must protect my body from the bad health effects.
To build a strong immune system and energy reserve in preparation for unexpected life events.
To model healthy behaviors for my family and the young people in my life....

Stress! Protect Your Body From Stress Effects!

Decrease Stress Vulnerability

- Do some type of exercise every day and consume a healthy diet most of the time.

- Do not abuse substances like tobacco, alcohol, or drugs.

- Surround yourself with positive people and friends you can count on in times of crisis.

- Get plenty of sleep...zzzzzzzzzzzzzzzzzzzzzzzzzzzzzzzz!

- Become a great communicator!

- Get organized or at least have a plan for work, family, money, etc.

- Simplify, prioritize and create shared expectations with family and co-workers

- Take time to laugh, add humor to home and work situations, and have some fun every day.

- Nurture the spiritual components in your life.

- Share your life with a "significant other" - someone who is truly your soul mate.

Fitness

Accumulate at least 30 minutes of at least moderate intensity physical activity each day.

- Walking/Swimming/Biking/Any General Aerobic Activity

- The equivalent of walking 1.5 miles at 3 to 4 m.p.h.

- Can be broken up into several segments of 10 or 15 minutes

- Higher intensity workouts may give you even more health benefits but may increase injury risk.

Strengthen muscles to maintain lean body mass, increase metabolism, support your skeleton, and prevent osteoporosis.

- Use weights, bands, or calisthenics. Three times per week/alternate days

- Do one set of 8 to 12 repetitions. When 8 is easy, go up to 10, when 10 is easy, go up to 12, when 12 is easy go up on your weight or resistance and go back to 8 repetitions.

- Always include: Abdominals, Hamstrings, Upper Back, Lower Back

- If you have extra time: Quadriceps, Pectorals, Inner Thighs, Outer Thighs, Biceps, Triceps,

Stretch each muscle group to maintain function and flexibility.

- The best time to stretch is when you are warm (after aerobic exercise or a hot shower or bath).

- Do not stretch when your muscles are cold!

- Enjoy Pilates or Yoga to increase flexibility but modify for individual differences.

- Attention Weekend Warriors!!! Prepare for Intense Work, Lifting or Sports: Before golf, tennis, yard work, lifting, etc. warm-up until you have a light sweat, do general stretches, and then go through the movements specific to the activity (without the equipment). Example: perform a golf swing without the club.

Nutrition

ANTI-OXIDIZE with Fruits and Vegetables!

- Eat 5 or more different raw fruits each day. Include many colors, the skin, and other fibers.

- Eat 5 or more raw, non-starchy vegetables each day. Include many colors, raw if possible.

- If you have difficulty eating this many, add Juice Plus+ whole-food product.

- Include a maximum of 2 servings of grains, breads and cereals (zero if you are trying to lose weight). Try sprouted breads, high-fiber, whole grain cereals and pasta, or brown rice.

Chose healthy fats!

- Choose your 30-60 grams/day wisely. Use canola oil, flaxseed oil, or olive oil.

- Increase Omega 3 fatty acids (wild fish, flax seeds, walnuts, grass-fed meat, omega-3 rich eggs)

- Avoid all foods that say "partially-hydrogenated fat"

- Avoid corn oil and safflower oil to improve omega-6 to omega-3 ratios

- Include healthy fats like nuts, seeds, salmon(wild), and avocados.

- Protect fatty acids with antioxidants (leafy greens, almonds, hazelnuts, Juice Plus+)

- Choose a high quality fish oil supplement if you do not consume enough fish

Choose healthy protein sources...

- Avoid consuming too much protein of any kind.

- Choose lean cuts of meat, chicken (free range if possible) or wild fish.

- Soy Products, organic milk or cheese, eggs from free range hens

- Lentils, beans or small handful of raw nuts or seeds.

Increase Fiber - Scrub away carcinogens!

- Include 20-30 grams of fiber in your diet per day (fruits, veggies, grains, whole grain flours and baked goods, beans, peas, nuts, seeds, Juice Plus+ thins)

Stay Hydrated!

- Drink plenty of water during the day. Caffeine drinks do not count.

- Try adding lemon or lime juice or try seltzer water with a little fruit juice added.

You health nuts are going to feel really stupid some day lying in a hospital bed dying of nothing.

Redd Foxx

Appendix 1

THE FIVE MINUTE STRETCH

Follow this sequence for a safe, efficient, flexibility workout. Remember to warm-up before you start, hold each position for at least 10-15 seconds and do not bounce. Close your eyes, take a few deep breaths and clear your mind. This is your time to relax.

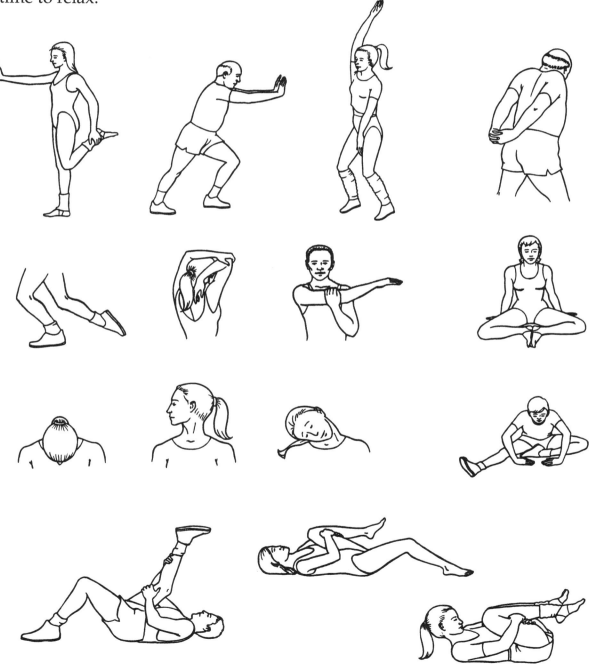

Notes

Health and Fitness Assessment Profile

This chart provides a place for you to keep track of the important numbers that impact your health. Your physician and personal trainer can help you measure these parameters before and after your lifestyle changes.

Name_____ Start Date_____

Sex M/F   Height_____(inches) Date of Birth_____

Critical Health Marker	Pre-Test Data	Goal	Post Test 1	Post Test 2
Resting Heart Rate (bts/min)				
Weight/lbs				
Body Mass Index (kg/m2)				
Circumference/Chest (in)				
Circumference/Waist (in)				
Circumference/Hips (in)				
Circumference/Thigh (in)				
Body Fat Percentage Measured by_____				
Aerobic Capacity Type of Test_____				
Flexibility Type of Test_____				
Abdominal Strength Type of Test_____				

Critical Health Marker	Pre-Test Data	Goal	Post Test 1	Post Test 2
Posture Analysis				
Smoking Status				
Depression Test				
Blood Pressure/Systolic				
Blood Pressure/Diastolic				
Blood Data				
Cholesterol/Total				
Cholesterol/LDL				
Cholesterol/HDL				
Triglycerides				
Homocysteine				
C-Reactive Protein				
Fibrinogen				
Fasting Glucose				
Serum phytochemicals				
Beta-carotene				
Alpha-carotene				
Lutein/zeaxanthin				
Lycopene				
Alpha-tocopherol				

Notes or Other
Measurements_____
_____
_____
_____
_____
_____

Appendix 3

Wellness From Within Journal

The only reason I'd take up jogging is so I could hear heavy breathing again.
Erma Bombeck

Fitness Challenges_____

_____

Goals and Solutions_____

_____

_____

_____

_____

Never eat more than you can lift.
Miss Piggy

Nutrition Challenges_____

_____

Goals and Solutions_____

_____

_____

_____

_____

> *Death is nature's way of telling us to slow down.*
> Woody Allen

Stress Management Challenges_____

_____

Goals and Solutions_____

_____

_____

_____

_____

> *Face your deficiencies and acknowledge them; but do not let them master you. Let them teach you patience, sweetness, insight....When we do the best we can, we never know what miracle is wrought in our life, or in the life of another.*
> Helen Keller

Attitude Challenges_____

_____

Goals and Solutions_____

_____

_____

_____

_____

> *Lost time is never found again.*
> Benjamin Franklin   1748

Time Management Challenges_____

_____

Goals and Solutions_____

_____

_____

_____

_____

> *Two are better than one, because they have a good return for their work: If one falls down, his friend can help him up. But pity the man who falls and has no one to help him up!*
> Ecclesiastes 4:9-10

Support System Challenges_____

_____

Goals and Solutions_____

_____

_____

_____

FOUR DAY FOOD JOURNAL

Write down everything you eat for four days. This really means everything. Try to eat normally and avoid changing your habits. Be sure to include beverages, condiments, gum, candy, salad dressings, etc. Record what you eat, when you eat it, and why. Was it hunger? Was it emotional stress, anxiety, or boredom? What are the approximate number of calories? Research shows that journaling your intake gives you more control and helps you successfully achieve your nutrition and weight loss goals. A nutrition professional can help you look for places to improve and make substitutions.

Day and Date_____				
Food Eaten	When/Where	With Whom	Why?	Calories

Day and Date_____				
Food Eaten	When/Where	With Whom	Why?	Calories

Day and Date_____

Food Eaten	When/Where	With Whom	Why?	Calories

Day and Date_____

Food Eaten	When/Where	With Whom	Why?	Calories

Appendix 5

Personal Wellness Plan

Name _____ Date_____

Age _____ Sex _____ Height _____' _____" Weight _____ lbs

General Wellness Goals _____

_____

_____

Body Fat:_____% 6 month goal _____% 1 year goal _____%

Exercise Plan

Fitness Goals _____

_____

_____

Cardiovascular Fitness (see Chapter Four)

Activity: Circle activities that you like and that will fit into your lifestyle.

Walking	Road Cycling	Swimming	Low-impact Aerobics
Jogging	Stationary Cycling	Aqua-Aerobics	High-impact Aerobics
Stair Climbing	Cross Country Skiing	Step Aerobics	Other _____

Frequency _____ days/week

Duration _____ minutes within my Target Heart Zone

Intensity _____ % of Maximal Heart Rate Reserve

    Target Heart Rate Zone _____ beats/min to _____ beats/min

    In 6 seconds _____ to _____

Use Rating of Perceived Exertion Scale

Muscular Strength and Endurance _____ days/ week

Mode of resistance   calisthenics   light weights

                         stretchy bands   heavy weights

Include the following muscles and muscle groups: _____

_____

_____

_____

Perform _____ sets of_____ repetitions.

Choose a resistance such that you feel fatigue on the last 3-4 repetitions.

Flexibility _____ days/week

Perform slow, static stretching.

Hold each position 10-30 seconds.

Warm-up prior to stretching.

_____

_____

_____

Nutrition Plan

Nutrition Goals_____

_____

_____

My ideal weight is _____ lbs.

Stress Plan

Stress Management Goals _____

_____

_____

_____

TOTAL WORKOUT LOG

	Example							
Date	5/2/89							
Circulatory Warm-up& Stretch	✓							
Type of Aerobic Activity *	W							
Minutes of Aerobic Activity	20							
Abdominals	2/15							
Upper Back	2/8/B							
Chest	2/10/60							
Hamstrings	2/10/30							
Biceps	2/10/B							
Triceps	2/10/B							
Deltoids	2/10/B							
Final Stretch and Relaxation	✓							

Muscle Strength and Endurance ** (Abdominals – Deltoids)

Aerobic Activity In THZ (Chest, Hamstrings)

* W = Walk   S = Swim
J = Jog   A = Aerobic Dance
C = Cycle   O = Other

** Sets/Repetitions/Resistance
(e.g., 2/10/25 = 2 sets of 10 repetitions with 25 pounds)
(e.g., 2/10/B = 2 sets of 10 repetitions with a stretchy band).

Notes

Recommended Resources

Author Information: Toni Tickel Branner, M.A.

Professional Speaking, Workshops, and Seminars, Fitness Tips and Recipes
The Safe Exercise Handbook with upper body & lower body exercise bands
Information on *Wilby's Fitness Book* for children,
Website: www.tonibranner.com
email: tonibranner@aol.com   Phone: (704)551-9051

To buy more copies of this book (It comes with or without the two bands)
The Safe Exercise Handbook, 5th Edition (www.kendallhunt.com or 1-800-228-0810)

Recommended Books

The Omega-3 Connection by Andrew L. Stoll, M.D.
Health Basics by Michael S. Richardson, M.D. (www.nextdecade.com)
Take a Load Off Your Heart by Joseph C. Piscatella and Barry A. Franklin
Dr. Sears' LEAN Kids by William Sears, M.D. and Peter Sears, M.D.
Wilby's Fitness Book (www.tonibranner.com)
Intuitive Eating by Humbart Santillo, N.D., Ph.D. (800-381-2700)

Recommended Websites and Newsletters

Nutrition Action (newsletter)   *www.cspinet.org*
Tufts Newsletter   *www.healthletter.tufts.edu*
American Council on Exercise   *www.acefitness.org*
American Heart Association   *www.americanheart.org*
American Dietetic Association   *www.eatright.org*
American College of Sports Medicine   *www.acsm.org*
American College of Cardiology   *www.acc.org*
American Cancer Society   *www.cancer.org*

Product Recommendations

Fitness Equipment
For fairly priced, high quality fitness equipment, weights, mats, stability balls, videos, etc.
Fitness Wholesale: 1-888-FW-ORDER or fitnesswholesale.com

For Juice Plus+® Whole Food Nutrition Products
17 Fruits and Vegetables available in Capsules, Chewables, or Gummies
For information and research reprints
Go to: *www.juiceplus.com* Or Call 1-800-347-6350